2. Quinoa and Black Bean Salad

Ingredient:

• 1 cup uncooked quinoa, rinsed
• 1 (15 oz) can black beans, rinsed and drained
• 1 cup diced cucumber
• 1 cup diced tomatoes
• 1/2 cup diced red onion
• 1/4 cup chopped fresh cilantro
• 2 tbsp lime juice
• 1 tbsp olive oil
• 1 tsp ground cumin
• 1/2 tsp chili powder
• Salt and pepper to taste

Instructions:

1. Cook the quinoa according to package instructions. Allow to cool completely.

2. In a large bowl, combine the cooked quinoa, black beans, cucumber, tomatoes, red onion, and cilantro.

3. In a small bowl, whisk together the lime juice, olive oil, cumin, and chili powder. Season with salt and pepper.

4. Pour the dressing over the quinoa and bean mixture and toss to coat evenly.

5. Refrigerate for at least 30 minutes to allow the flavors to meld.

6. Serve chilled or at room temperature.

This quinoa and black bean salad is a great option for young men aiming for weight loss. Quinoa is a high•protein, high•fiber grain that can help keep you feeling full, while the black beans provide additional protein and fiber. The vegetables add nutrients and volume to the salad without a lot of calories. The simple lime•cumin dressing adds flavor without a lot of extra fat or sugar. This makes for a satisfying and nutritious meal or side dish.

3. Baked Salmon with Asparagus

Ingredient:

- 4 (6 oz) salmon fillets
- 1 lb asparagus, trimmed
- 2 tbsp olive oil
- 2 tsp lemon juice
- 1 tsp garlic powder
- 1 tsp dried dill
- Salt and pepper to taste

Instructions:

1. Preheat oven to 400°F. Line a baking sheet with parchment paper.

2. Place the salmon fillets and asparagus spears on the prepared baking sheet. Drizzle with olive oil and lemon juice, then sprinkle with garlic powder, dried dill, salt, and pepper.

3. Bake for 12•15 minutes, or until the salmon is cooked through and flakes easily with a fork, and the asparagus is tender•crisp.

4. Serve the baked salmon immediately, with the roasted asparagus on the side.

This baked salmon and asparagus dish is an excellent choice for young men aiming for weight loss for a few reasons:

1. Salmon is a lean, high•protein fish that is rich in healthy omega•3 fatty acids, which can help support weight loss and overall health.

2. Asparagus is a low•calorie, high•fiber vegetable that can help you feel full and satisfied.

3. The dish is baked rather than fried, which keeps the calorie and fat content low.

4. The simple seasoning of lemon, garlic, and dill adds flavor without the need for heavy sauces or dressings.

This meal is nutritious, filling, and easy to prepare, making it a great option for young men focused on weight loss.

Welcome to ***"Cookbook for Weight Loss Young Men: Tasty, Low-Calorie Dishes to Boost Your Weight Loss Journey."*** This cookbook is crafted specifically for young men who are eager to embark on a healthier lifestyle without sacrificing the joy of eating delicious meals. Whether you're new to cooking or a seasoned chef, this collection of over 110 recipes is designed to simplify your weight loss journey with flavorful, easy-to-make dishes that will keep you motivated and satisfied.

As a young man, balancing the demands of school, work, social life, and fitness can be challenging. Often, the convenience of fast food and unhealthy snacks becomes tempting, making it harder to maintain a healthy diet. This book aims to change that by offering recipes that are not only nutritious and low in calories but also quick to prepare, ensuring you can fit healthy eating into your busy schedule.

Each recipe in this cookbook is carefully curated to provide the essential nutrients your body needs while keeping the calorie count low. You'll find a variety of options, from hearty breakfasts and protein-packed lunches to satisfying dinners and guilt-free desserts. These meals are designed to fuel your workouts, support muscle growth, and promote fat loss, helping you achieve your weight loss goals without feeling deprived.

In addition to the recipes, you'll find useful tips on meal prepping, grocery shopping, and maintaining a balanced diet. We've also included nutritional information for each dish, so you can keep track of your intake and make informed choices about what you're eating.

Cooking healthy meals doesn't have to be complicated or time-consuming. With this cookbook, you'll discover how easy and enjoyable it can be to prepare tasty, low-calorie dishes that support your weight loss journey. So, grab your apron, fire up the stove, and get ready to transform your diet and your body with these delicious recipes. Let's get cooking!

1. Grilled Chicken Salad

Ingredient:

• 4 boneless, skinless chicken breasts
• 1 tbsp olive oil
• 1 tsp garlic powder
• 1 tsp dried oregano
• Salt and pepper to taste
• 8 cups mixed greens (spinach, romaine, arugula, etc.)
• 1 cup cherry tomatoes, halved
• 1/2 cucumber, sliced
• 1/4 red onion, thinly sliced
• 2 tbsp balsamic vinegar
• 1 tbsp Dijon mustard

Instructions:

1. Preheat grill or grill pan to medium·high heat.

2. Rub the chicken breasts with olive oil and season with garlic powder, oregano, salt, and pepper.

3. Grill the chicken for 5·7 minutes per side, or until cooked through. Allow to rest for 5 minutes, then slice or shred the chicken.

4. In a large salad bowl, combine the mixed greens, tomatoes, cucumber, and red onion.

5. In a small bowl, whisk together the balsamic vinegar and Dijon mustard. Drizzle the dressing over the salad and toss to coat.

6. Top the salad with the grilled chicken.

This salad is packed with lean protein from the grilled chicken, and the vegetables provide fiber, vitamins, and minerals. The balsamic vinaigrette dressing adds flavor without a lot of extra calories or fat. This makes for a filling and nutritious meal that can support weight loss goals.

4. Turkey and Spinach Wrap

Ingredient:

• 4 whole wheat tortillas or wraps
• 8 oz sliced turkey breast
• 2 cups fresh spinach leaves
• 1/2 cup shredded carrots
• 1/4 cup sliced cucumber
• 2 tbsp hummus
• 1 tbsp Dijon mustard
• Salt and pepper to taste

Instructions:

1. Lay the tortillas or wraps out on a clean surface.

2. Divide the turkey slices evenly among the tortillas, placing them in the center.

3. Top the turkey with the spinach leaves, shredded carrots, and sliced cucumber.

4. In a small bowl, mix together the hummus and Dijon mustard. Spread this mixture evenly over the fillings on each wrap.

5. Season with salt and pepper to taste.

6. Fold the bottom of the tortilla up over the filling, then fold in the sides and continue rolling tightly into a wrap. Slice the wraps in half diagonally and serve.

This turkey and spinach wrap is a great option for young men aiming for weight loss for several reasons:

1. Turkey is a lean, high•protein meat that can help keep you feeling full and satisfied.
2. Spinach is a nutrient•dense leafy green that provides fiber, vitamins, and minerals.
3. The addition of carrots and cucumber adds crunchy texture and more nutrients.
4. The hummus and Dijon mustard provide flavor without a lot of extra calories or fat.
5. Whole wheat tortillas are a complex carbohydrate that can help provide sustained energy.

This wrap is easy to prepare, portable, and packed with nutrients to support a healthy weight loss journey.

5. Greek Yogurt with Berries

Ingredient:

• 1 cup plain Greek yogurt
• 1 cup mixed berries (such as blueberries, raspberries, and/or blackberries)
• 1 tbsp honey (optional)

Instructions:

1. Scoop the Greek yogurt into a bowl or serving dish.
2. Top the yogurt with the mixed berries.
3. If desired, drizzle the honey over the top of the berries.

That's it! This healthy snack or light meal is incredibly simple to prepare but provides a lot of nutritional benefits:

• Greek yogurt is high in protein, which can help keep you feeling full and satisfied.

• Berries are packed with fiber, vitamins, and antioxidants, making them a nutrient•dense choice.

• Honey can add a touch of sweetness if desired, but is optional.

This Greek yogurt and berry parfait is a great option for young men aiming for weight loss for a few reasons:

1. It's low in calories but high in nutrients and protein to support weight management.

2. The combination of protein, fiber, and natural sugars from the berries can help curb cravings and provide sustained energy.

3. It's quick and easy to prepare, making it a convenient healthy snack or light meal.

4. The versatility of the ingredients allows for different flavor combinations to keep it interesting.

Overall, this simple Greek yogurt and berry dish is a nutritious and satisfying choice for young men focused on weight loss.

6. Egg White Omelette with Vegetables

Ingredient:

• 4 egg whites
• 1 tbsp olive oil
• 1/2 cup diced bell pepper
• 1/2 cup diced onion
• 1 cup spinach leaves, chopped
• 2 tbsp shredded low•fat cheddar cheese (optional)
• Salt and pepper to taste

Instructions:

1. Crack the egg whites into a small bowl and whisk lightly with a fork.

2. Heat the olive oil in a non•stick skillet over medium heat.

3. Add the diced bell pepper and onion to the skillet and sauté for 2•3 minutes until softened.

4. Pour the egg whites into the skillet and let them sit for 30 seconds to a minute to set the bottom.

5. Use a spatula to gently push the cooked egg towards the center, tilting the pan to allow the uncooked egg to flow to the edges.

6. Once the eggs are mostly set, add the chopped spinach leaves and fold the omelette in half.

7. If using, sprinkle the shredded cheddar cheese over the top. Cook for an additional 1•2 minutes until the cheese is melted and the omelette is cooked through. Slide the omelette onto a plate and season with salt and pepper to taste.

This egg white omelette with vegetables is an excellent choice for young men aiming for weight loss for several reasons:

• Egg whites are low in calories but high in protein, which can help keep you feeling full.
• The vegetables add fiber, vitamins, and minerals without a lot of extra calories.
• The dish is cooked in a small amount of healthy olive oil rather than butter or other high•fat ingredients.
• The optional cheese provides a bit of creaminess and flavor without overdoing the calories or fat.

7. Grilled Shrimp Skewers

Ingredient:

- 1 lb large shrimp, peeled and deveined
- 2 tbsp olive oil
- 2 tbsp lemon juice
- 1 tsp garlic powder
- 1 tsp dried oregano
- 1/4 tsp red pepper flakes (optional)
- Salt and pepper to taste
- Wooden or metal skewers

Instructions:

1. In a medium bowl, combine the shrimp, olive oil, lemon juice, garlic powder, oregano, and red pepper flakes (if using). Toss to coat the shrimp evenly. Season with salt and pepper.
2. Thread the shrimp onto the skewers, leaving a small space between each one.
3. Preheat grill or grill pan to medium•high heat.
4. Grill the shrimp skewers for 2•3 minutes per side, or until the shrimp are opaque and cooked through.
5. Serve the grilled shrimp skewers immediately.

This grilled shrimp skewer recipe is an excellent choice for young men aiming for weight loss for a few reasons:

1. Shrimp is a lean, high•protein seafood that is low in calories and fat, making it a great protein source for weight loss.
2. The simple marinade of lemon, garlic, and herbs adds flavor without a lot of extra calories or sodium.
3. Grilling the shrimp keeps the cooking method light and healthy, rather than frying or sautéing.
4. Serving the shrimp on skewers makes for a fun, portable, and portion•controlled meal or snack.
5. The dish can be easily paired with a side salad or roasted vegetables for a complete, nutrient•dense meal.

Overall, these grilled shrimp skewers are a delicious and nutritious option that can support a young man's weight loss goals.

8. Zucchini Noodles with Pesto

Ingredient:

• 3 medium zucchinis, spiralized or julienned into noodles
• 1/2 cup basil pesto (store•bought or homemade)
• 1/4 cup cherry tomatoes, halved
• 2 tbsp toasted pine nuts
• 2 tbsp grated Parmesan cheese (optional)
• Salt and pepper to taste

Instructions:

1. Use a spiralizer, julienne peeler, or vegetable peeler to cut the zucchinis into long, thin noodles.

2. In a large bowl, toss the zucchini noodles with the basil pesto until the noodles are evenly coated.

3. Top the pesto•coated zucchini noodles with the cherry tomatoes, toasted pine nuts, and Parmesan cheese (if using).

4. Season with salt and pepper to taste. Serve immediately, or refrigerate for up to 3 days.

This zucchini noodle dish is an excellent choice for young men aiming for weight loss for several reasons:

1. Zucchini noodles are a low•calorie, low•carb alternative to traditional pasta, making them a great option for those watching their carb and calorie intake.

2. Basil pesto provides flavor and healthy fats from the olive oil and pine nuts, without a lot of added calories or sodium.

3. The cherry tomatoes add a pop of color, vitamins, and antioxidants.

4. The optional Parmesan cheese provides a creamy, savory element without overdoing the calories. The dish is easy to prepare and can be made ahead of time for a quick, healthy meal.

Overall, this zucchini noodle dish with pesto is a delicious and nutritious option that can support a young man's weight loss goals.

9. Lean Beef Stir•Fry with Broccoli

Ingredient:

• 1 lb lean beef (such as sirloin or flank steak), thinly sliced
• 2 tbsp low•sodium soy sauce
• 1 tbsp rice vinegar
• 1 tsp sesame oil
• 1 tsp cornstarch
• 2 cloves garlic, minced
• 1 tbsp grated fresh ginger
• 2 cups broccoli florets
• 1 red bell pepper, thinly sliced
• 1 cup sliced mushrooms
• 2 tbsp olive oil
• Salt and pepper to taste
• Cooked brown rice, for serving (optional)

Instructions:

1. In a medium bowl, combine the sliced beef, soy sauce, rice vinegar, sesame oil, and cornstarch. Toss to coat the beef and let marinate for 15 minutes.

2. Heat the olive oil in a large skillet or wok over high heat. Add the garlic and ginger and cook for 1 minute, until fragrant.

3. Add the marinated beef and stir•fry for 2•3 minutes, until the beef is mostly cooked through.

4. Add the broccoli, bell pepper, and mushrooms to the skillet. Stir•fry for an additional 3•4 minutes, until the vegetables are tender•crisp.

5. Season the stir•fry with salt and pepper to taste. Serve the beef and vegetable stir•fry over cooked brown rice, if desired.

This lean beef and broccoli stir•fry is an excellent choice for young men aiming for weight loss for several reasons:

1. Lean beef is a high•protein, nutrient•dense meat that can help keep you feeling full and satisfied.

2. Broccoli, bell peppers, and mushrooms are low•calorie, high•fiber vegetables that add volume and nutrients to the dish.

10. Chickpea and Tomato Salad

Ingredient:

- 1 (15 oz) can chickpeas, rinsed and drained
- 1 cup cherry tomatoes, halved
- 1/2 cup diced cucumber
- 1/4 cup diced red onion
- 2 tbsp chopped fresh parsley
- 2 tbsp lemon juice
- 1 tbsp olive oil
- 1 tsp Dijon mustard
- 1/4 tsp garlic powder
- Salt and pepper to taste

Instructions:

1. In a large bowl, combine the chickpeas, cherry tomatoes, cucumber, red onion, and parsley.

2. In a small bowl, whisk together the lemon juice, olive oil, Dijon mustard, and garlic powder. Season with salt and pepper.

3. Pour the dressing over the chickpea and vegetable mixture and toss gently to coat.

4. Refrigerate the salad for at least 30 minutes to allow the flavors to meld. Serve chilled or at room temperature.

This chickpea and tomato salad is an excellent choice for young men aiming for weight loss for several reasons:

1. Chickpeas are a high•protein, high•fiber legume that can help keep you feeling full and satisfied.

2. The fresh vegetables like tomatoes, cucumber, and onion add nutrients, fiber, and volume to the salad without a lot of calories.

3. The simple lemon•Dijon dressing provides flavor without relying on high•calorie or high•fat ingredients.

Overall, this chickpea and tomato salad is a nutritious, filling, and delicious option for young men focused on weight loss. The versatile ingredients can also be customized to individual tastes and preferences.

11. Spicy Tuna Salad

Ingredient:

• 2 (5 oz) cans of tuna, drained
• 2 tbsp plain Greek yogurt
• 1 tbsp Dijon mustard
• 1 tbsp hot sauce (such as Sriracha)
• 1 tbsp lemon juice
• 1/4 cup diced celery
• 2 tbsp diced red onion
• 2 tbsp chopped fresh parsley
• Salt and pepper to taste

Instructions:

1. In a medium bowl, combine the drained tuna, Greek yogurt, Dijon mustard, hot sauce, and lemon juice. Mix well until fully incorporated.

2. Fold in the diced celery, red onion, and chopped parsley. Season with salt and pepper to taste.

3. Serve the spicy tuna salad on a bed of mixed greens, stuffed into a tomato or avocado half, or scooped onto whole grain crackers or toast.

This spicy tuna salad is an excellent choice for young men aiming for weight loss for several reasons:

1. Tuna is a lean, high•protein seafood that is low in calories and fat, making it a great protein source for weight loss.

2. The Greek yogurt adds creaminess and extra protein without a lot of extra calories or fat.

3. The Dijon mustard and hot sauce provide bold flavor without relying on high•calorie condiments.

4. The fresh vegetables like celery and onion add crunch, fiber, and nutrients. The overall dish is low in calories but high in protein, which can help keep you feeling full and satisfied.

This spicy tuna salad can be enjoyed on its own, as a sandwich or wrap filling, or as a topping for a salad. It's a versatile and nutritious option for young men focused on weight loss.

12. Lentil Soup

Ingredient:

• 1 tbsp olive oil
• 1 onion, diced
• 3 cloves garlic, minced
• 2 carrots, peeled and diced
• 2 celery stalks, diced
• 1 cup dried brown or green lentils, rinsed
• 6 cups low•sodium vegetable or chicken broth
• 1 (14.5 oz) can diced tomatoes
• 2 tsp dried thyme
• 1 tsp dried oregano
• Salt and pepper to taste
• Chopped parsley for garnish (optional)

Instructions:

1. In a large pot or Dutch oven, heat the olive oil over medium heat. Add the onion and sauté for 3•4 minutes until translucent.

2. Add the garlic, carrots, and celery. Sauté for an additional 2•3 minutes.

3. Stir in the lentils, broth, diced tomatoes, thyme, and oregano. Season with salt and pepper.

4. Bring the soup to a boil, then reduce heat and let simmer for 20•25 minutes, or until the lentils are tender.

5. Taste and adjust seasoning as needed. Serve the lentil soup hot, garnished with chopped parsley if desired.

This lentil soup is an excellent choice for young men aiming for weight loss for several reasons:

1. Lentils are a high•protein, high•fiber legume that can help keep you feeling full and satisfied.

2. The vegetables, including onions, carrots, and celery, add fiber, vitamins, and minerals without a lot of extra calories.

13. Chicken and Vegetable Stir•Fry

Ingredient:

• 1 lb boneless, skinless chicken breasts, cut into 1•inch pieces
• 2 tbsp low•sodium soy sauce
• 1 tbsp rice vinegar
• 1 tsp sesame oil
• 1 tbsp cornstarch
• 2 tbsp olive oil
• 3 cloves garlic, minced
• 1 tbsp grated fresh ginger
• 1 red bell pepper, sliced
• 1 cup broccoli florets
• 1 cup sliced mushrooms
• 1 cup snow peas or snap peas
• 2 green onions, sliced
• Salt and pepper to taste
• Cooked brown rice, for serving (optional)

Instructions:

1. In a medium bowl, combine the chicken, soy sauce, rice vinegar, sesame oil, and cornstarch. Toss to coat the chicken and let marinate for 15 minutes.

2. Heat the olive oil in a large skillet or wok over high heat. Add the garlic and ginger and cook for 1 minute, until fragrant.

3. Add the marinated chicken to the skillet and stir•fry for 3•4 minutes, until the chicken is mostly cooked through.

4. Add the bell pepper, broccoli, mushrooms, and snow peas to the skillet. Stir•fry for an additional 4•5 minutes, until the vegetables are tender•crisp.

5. Remove the skillet from heat and stir in the sliced green onions. Season with salt and pepper to taste. Serve the chicken and vegetable stir•fry over cooked brown rice, if desired.

Overall, this chicken and vegetable stir•fry is a delicious and nutritious option that can support a young man's weight loss goals.

14. Turkey Meatballs with Zucchini Noodles

Ingredient:

• 1 lb ground turkey
• 1/2 cup whole wheat breadcrumbs
• 1 egg, lightly beaten
• 2 tbsp grated Parmesan cheese
• 2 cloves garlic, minced
• 1 tsp dried oregano
• 1/2 tsp salt
• 1/4 tsp black pepper
• 3 medium zucchinis, spiralized or julienned into noodles
• 1 cup marinara sauce

Instructions:

1. Preheat oven to 400°F. Line a baking sheet with parchment paper.

2. In a large bowl, combine the ground turkey, breadcrumbs, egg, Parmesan, garlic, oregano, salt, and pepper. Mix until well incorporated.

3. Roll the turkey mixture into 1•inch meatballs and place them on the prepared baking sheet.

4. Bake the meatballs for 18•20 minutes, or until cooked through.

5. While the meatballs are baking, prepare the zucchini noodles.

6. In a large skillet, heat the marinara sauce over medium heat. Add the zucchini noodles and toss to coat.

7. Cook the zucchini noodles for 2•3 minutes, just until they start to soften. Serve the turkey meatballs over the zucchini noodles, with the marinara sauce.

This turkey meatball and zucchini noodle dish is an excellent choice for young men aiming for weight loss for several reasons:

1. Ground turkey is a lean protein that is lower in fat and calories compared to ground beef.
2. Zucchini noodles are a low•calorie, low•carb alternative to traditional pasta, making them a great option for those watching their carb intake.

15. Cauliflower Rice with Grilled Chicken

Ingredient:

• 1 head of cauliflower, riced (about 4 cups riced cauliflower)
• 2 boneless, skinless chicken breasts
• 1 tbsp olive oil
• 1 tsp garlic powder
• 1 tsp dried oregano
• Salt and pepper to taste
• 2 tbsp chopped fresh parsley

Instructions:

1. Preheat grill or grill pan to medium•high heat.

2. Rub the chicken breasts with 1 tsp of the olive oil and season with garlic powder, oregano, salt, and pepper.

3. Grill the chicken for 5•7 minutes per side, or until cooked through. Allow to rest for 5 minutes, then slice or shred the chicken.

4. While the chicken is cooking, heat the remaining 1 tsp of olive oil in a large skillet over medium heat.

5. Add the riced cauliflower to the skillet and sauté for 5•7 minutes, stirring occasionally, until the cauliflower is tender.

6. Remove the cauliflower rice from heat and stir in the chopped parsley.

7. Serve the grilled chicken on top of the cauliflower rice.

This cauliflower rice and grilled chicken dish is an excellent choice for young men aiming for weight loss for several reasons:

1. Cauliflower rice is a low•calorie, low•carb alternative to traditional rice, making it a great option for those watching their carb and calorie intake.

2. Grilled chicken is a lean, high•protein protein source that can help keep you feeling full and satisfied.

3. The simple seasoning of garlic, oregano, salt, and pepper adds flavor without a lot of extra calories or sodium

16. Spaghetti Squash with Marinara Sauce

Ingredient:

• 1 medium spaghetti squash, halved lengthwise and seeds removed
• 1 tbsp olive oil
• 1 (24 oz) jar marinara sauce
• 2 cloves garlic, minced
• 1 tsp dried oregano
• 1/4 tsp red pepper flakes (optional)
• Salt and pepper to taste
• Grated Parmesan cheese (optional)

Instructions:

1. Preheat oven to 400°F. Line a baking sheet with parchment paper.

2. Place the spaghetti squash halves cut•side down on the prepared baking sheet. Roast for 40•50 minutes, until the squash is tender and easily shreds with a fork.

3. Remove the spaghetti squash from the oven and let cool slightly. Use a fork to shred the flesh of the squash into spaghetti•like strands.

4. In a medium saucepan, combine the marinara sauce, garlic, oregano, and red pepper flakes (if using). Simmer over medium heat for 5•7 minutes, stirring occasionally.

5. Add the shredded spaghetti squash to the marinara sauce and toss to coat.

6. Season the spaghetti squash and marinara mixture with salt and pepper to taste.

7. Serve the spaghetti squash with marinara sauce, topped with grated Parmesan cheese if desired.

This spaghetti squash with marinara sauce is an excellent choice for young men aiming for weight loss for several reasons:

1. Spaghetti squash is a low•calorie, low•carb alternative to traditional pasta, making it a great option for those watching their carb and calorie Intake.

2. The marinara sauce provides flavor and nutrients without a lot of added sugar or fat.

3. The dish is easy to prepare and can be made ahead of time for a quick, healthy meal.

17. Baked Cod with Lemon and Dill

Ingredient:

- 4 (6 oz) cod fillets
- 2 tbsp olive oil
- 2 tbsp lemon juice
- 2 tsp dried dill
- 1 tsp garlic powder
- Salt and pepper to taste
- Lemon wedges for serving

Instructions:

1. Preheat oven to 400°F. Line a baking sheet with parchment paper.

2. Place the cod fillets on the prepared baking sheet.
3. In a small bowl, whisk together the olive oil, lemon juice, dried dill, and garlic powder.

4. Drizzle the lemon•dill mixture over the cod fillets, making sure to coat them evenly.

5. Season the cod with salt and pepper.

6. Bake for 12•15 minutes, or until the cod is opaque and flakes easily with a fork.

7. Serve the baked cod immediately, with lemon wedges on the side.

This baked cod with lemon and dill is an excellent choice for young men aiming for weight loss for several reasons:

1. Cod is a lean, high•protein fish that is low in calories and fat, making it a great protein source for weight loss.

2. The simple lemon and dill seasoning adds flavor without the need for heavy sauces or breading, keeping the dish light and healthy.

3. Baking the cod instead of frying keeps the cooking method low in calories and fat.

4. The dish is easy to prepare and can be made quickly, making it a convenient and nutritious meal option.

5. Cod is a versatile fish that can be paired with a variety of healthy side dishes, such as roasted vegetables or a fresh salad.

18. Grilled Turkey Burgers

Ingredient:

- 1 lb ground turkey
- 1/4 cup whole wheat breadcrumbs
- 1 egg, lightly beaten
- 2 tbsp finely chopped onion
- 1 tsp garlic powder
- 1 tsp dried oregano
- 1/2 tsp salt
- 1/4 tsp black pepper
- 4 whole wheat burger buns
- Toppings of your choice (such as lettuce, tomato, onion, pickles)

Instructions:

1. Preheat grill or grill pan to medium•high heat.

2. In a large bowl, combine the ground turkey, breadcrumbs, egg, onion, garlic powder, oregano, salt, and pepper. Mix until well incorporated.

3. Divide the turkey mixture into 4 equal portions and shape them into patties, about 1/2 inch thick.

4. Grill the turkey burgers for 4•5 minutes per side, or until cooked through and no longer pink in the center.

5. Toast the whole wheat buns on the grill for 1•2 minutes, if desired.

6. Serve the grilled turkey burgers on the toasted buns, topped with your desired toppings.

These grilled turkey burgers are an excellent choice for young men aiming for weight loss for several reasons:

1. Ground turkey is a lean protein that is lower in fat and calories compared to ground beef.

2. The whole wheat buns provide complex carbohydrates for sustained energy, without a lot of added sugar or refined flour.

3. The simple seasoning of garlic, oregano, salt, and pepper adds flavor without the need for high•calorie condiments or sauces.

19. Roasted Brussels Sprouts and Sweet Potatoes

Ingredient:

- 1 lb Brussels sprouts, trimmed and halved
- 2 medium sweet potatoes, peeled and cubed
- 2 tbsp olive oil
- 1 tsp garlic powder
- 1 tsp dried thyme
- 1/2 tsp salt
- 1/4 tsp black pepper

Instructions:

1. Preheat oven to 400°F. Line a large baking sheet with parchment paper.

2. In a large bowl, toss the Brussels sprouts and sweet potato cubes with the olive oil, garlic powder, thyme, salt, and pepper until evenly coated.

3. Spread the seasoned vegetables in a single layer on the prepared baking sheet.

4. Roast for 20•25 minutes, flipping the vegetables halfway through, until the Brussels sprouts are tender and lightly browned and the sweet potatoes are fork•tender. Serve the roasted Brussels sprouts and sweet potatoes warm.

This roasted Brussels sprouts and sweet potato dish is an excellent choice for young men aiming for weight loss for several reasons:

1. Brussels sprouts and sweet potatoes are both nutrient•dense, high•fiber vegetables that are low in calories.

2. The combination of the two vegetables provides a variety of vitamins, minerals, and antioxidants to support overall health.

3. Roasting the vegetables brings out their natural sweetness and caramelized flavors without the need for added fats or sugars.

4. The simple seasoning of garlic, thyme, salt, and pepper adds flavor without a lot of extra calories. This dish is easy to prepare and can be served as a side or as part of a larger meal.

Overall, this roasted Brussels sprouts and sweet potato recipe is a delicious and nutritious option that can support a young man's weight loss goals. The high•fiber, low•calorie vegetables provide a filling and satisfying side dish or meal component.

20. Vegetable and Tofu Stir•Fry

Ingredient:
- 1 block (14 oz) extra•firm tofu, pressed and cubed
- 2 tbsp low•sodium soy sauce
- 1 tbsp rice vinegar
- 1 tsp sesame oil
- 1 tbsp cornstarch
- 2 tbsp olive oil
- 3 cloves garlic, minced
- 1 tbsp grated fresh ginger
- 1 red bell pepper, sliced
- 1 cup broccoli florets
- 1 cup sliced mushrooms
- 1 cup snow peas or snap peas
- 2 green onions, sliced
- Salt and pepper to taste
- Cooked brown rice, for serving (optional)

Instructions:

1. In a medium bowl, combine the cubed tofu, soy sauce, rice vinegar, sesame oil, and cornstarch. Toss to coat the tofu and let marinate for 15 minutes.

2. Heat the olive oil in a large skillet or wok over high heat. Add the garlic and ginger and cook for 1 minute, until fragrant.

3. Add the marinated tofu to the skillet and stir•fry for 3•4 minutes, until the tofu is lightly browned.

4. Add the bell pepper, broccoli, mushrooms, and snow peas to the skillet. Stir•fry for an additional 4•5 minutes, until the vegetables are tender•crisp.

5. Remove the skillet from heat and stir in the sliced green onions. Season with salt and pepper to taste. Serve the vegetable and tofu stir•fry over cooked brown rice, if desired.

This vegetable and tofu stir•fry is an excellent choice for young men aiming for weight loss for several reasons:

1. Tofu is a plant•based, high•protein ingredient that is low in calories and fat, making it a great option for those watching their weight.

2. The variety of vegetables, including bell peppers, broccoli, mushrooms, and snow peas, provide fiber, vitamins, and minerals without a lot of extra calories.

21. Greek Salad with Grilled Chicken

Ingredient:

- 4 (6 oz) boneless, skinless chicken breasts
- 1 tbsp olive oil
- 1 tsp dried oregano
- Salt and pepper to taste
- 8 cups mixed greens (romaine, spinach, arugula, etc.)
- 1 cup cherry tomatoes, halved
- 1/2 cucumber, sliced
- 1/4 red onion, thinly sliced
- 1/2 cup crumbled feta cheese
- 1/4 cup pitted kalamata olives, halved
- 2 tbsp red wine vinegar
- 1 tbsp lemon juice
- 1 tbsp olive oil
- 1 tsp Dijon mustard
- 1 tsp dried oregano
- Salt and pepper to taste

Instructions:

1. Preheat grill or grill pan to medium•high heat.

2. Rub the chicken breasts with 1 tbsp olive oil and season with 1 tsp dried oregano, salt, and pepper.

3. Grill the chicken for 5•7 minutes per side, or until cooked through. Allow to rest for 5 minutes, then slice or chop the chicken.

4. In a large salad bowl, combine the mixed greens, cherry tomatoes, cucumber, red onion, feta cheese, and kalamata olives.

5. In a small bowl, whisk together the red wine vinegar, lemon juice, 1 tbsp olive oil, Dijon mustard, 1 tsp dried oregano, salt, and pepper.

6. Drizzle the dressing over the salad and toss to coat. Top the salad with the grilled chicken.

Overall, this Greek salad with grilled chicken is a delicious and nutritious option that can support a young man's weight loss goals.

22. Baked Chicken Breast with Green Beans

Ingredient:

• 4 (6 oz) boneless, skinless chicken breasts
• 1 tbsp olive oil
• 1 tsp garlic powder
• 1 tsp dried oregano
• 1/2 tsp salt
• 1/4 tsp black pepper
• 1 lb fresh green beans, trimmed
• 1 tbsp lemon juice

Instructions:
1. Preheat oven to 400°F. Line a baking sheet with parchment paper.

2. Place the chicken breasts on the prepared baking sheet. Drizzle with the olive oil and sprinkle with the garlic powder, oregano, salt, and pepper. Rub the seasoning all over the chicken.

3. Arrange the green beans around the chicken on the baking sheet.

4. Bake for 20•25 minutes, or until the chicken is cooked through and the green beans are tender•crisp.

5. Remove the baking sheet from the oven and drizzle the lemon juice over the green beans.

6. Serve the baked chicken breast immediately, with the lemon•garlic green beans on the side.

This baked chicken breast with green beans dish is an excellent choice for young men aiming for weight loss for several reasons:

1. Boneless, skinless chicken breasts are a lean, high•protein protein source that is low in calories and fat.

2. Green beans are a low•calorie, high•fiber vegetable that provides essential vitamins and minerals.

3. The simple seasoning of garlic, oregano, salt, and pepper adds flavor without the need for heavy sauces or breading.

23. Sautéed Kale with Garlic and Lemon

Ingredient:

- 1 lb kale, stems removed and leaves chopped
- 1 tbsp olive oil
- 3 cloves garlic, minced
- 2 tbsp lemon juice
- 1/4 tsp red pepper flakes (optional)
- Salt and pepper to taste

Instructions:

1. In a large skillet or wok, heat the olive oil over medium heat.

2. Add the minced garlic and sauté for 1 minute, until fragrant.

3. Add the chopped kale to the skillet and sauté for 3•5 minutes, stirring frequently, until the kale is wilted and tender.

4. Remove the skillet from heat and stir in the lemon juice. If using, add the red pepper flakes.

5. Season the sautéed kale with salt and pepper to taste.

6. Serve the kale warm, as a side dish or mixed into other meals.

This sautéed kale with garlic and lemon is an excellent choice for young men aiming for weight loss for several reasons:

1. Kale is a nutrient•dense, low•calorie leafy green that is high in fiber, vitamins, and minerals.

2. The simple preparation of sautéing the kale with garlic and lemon keeps the dish light and healthy, without the need for heavy sauces or seasonings.

3. The lemon juice adds a bright, tangy flavor to the kale without adding any extra calories.

Overall, this sautéed kale with garlic and lemon is a delicious and nutritious side dish or addition to a meal that can support a young man's weight loss goals. The combination of nutrient•dense kale and simple, flavorful seasonings makes it a great option for those looking to incorporate more vegetables into their diet.

24. Cottage Cheese with Pineapple

Ingredient:

• 1 cup low•fat or non•fat cottage cheese
• 1/2 cup diced fresh pineapple
• 1 tsp honey (optional)

Instructions:

1. In a small bowl, combine the cottage cheese and diced pineapple.

2. If desired, drizzle the honey over the top of the cottage cheese and pineapple mixture.

3. Stir gently to combine.

4. Serve immediately.

This cottage cheese and pineapple dish is an excellent choice for young men aiming for weight loss for several reasons:

1. Cottage cheese is a high•protein, low•fat dairy product that can help keep you feeling full and satisfied.

2. Pineapple is a low•calorie, high•fiber fruit that adds natural sweetness and nutrients to the dish.

3. The optional honey provides a touch of sweetness without a lot of added sugar.

4. The dish is incredibly simple to prepare, making it a convenient and healthy snack or light meal.

5. The combination of protein, fiber, and natural sugars can help curb cravings and provide sustained energy.

Overall, this cottage cheese and pineapple dish is a nutritious and delicious option that can support a young man's weight loss goals. It's a versatile snack or meal that can be enjoyed on its own or paired with other healthy foods.

25. Broiled Tilapia with Steamed Broccoli

Ingredient:

• 4 (6 oz) tilapia fillets
• 2 tbsp lemon juice
• 1 tsp olive oil
• 1 tsp garlic powder
• 1 tsp dried parsley
• Salt and pepper to taste
• 1 lb broccoli florets
• 2 tbsp water

Instructions:

1. Preheat the broiler and line a baking sheet with foil.

2. Place the tilapia fillets on the prepared baking sheet. Drizzle with lemon juice and olive oil, then sprinkle with garlic powder, dried parsley, salt, and pepper.

3. Broil the tilapia for 8•10 minutes, flipping halfway through, until the fish is opaque and flakes easily with a fork.

4. While the tilapia is broiling, place the broccoli florets in a microwave•safe bowl. Add the 2 tbsp of water, cover, and microwave for 3•4 minutes, until the broccoli is tender•crisp.

5. Drain any excess water from the broccoli. Serve the broiled tilapia fillets immediately, with the steamed broccoli on the side.

This broiled tilapia and steamed broccoli dish is an excellent choice for young men aiming for weight loss for several reasons:

1. Tilapia is a lean, white fish that is low in calories and fat, making it a great protein source for weight loss.

2. Broccoli is a low•calorie, high•fiber vegetable that provides essential vitamins, minerals, and antioxidants.

3. The simple seasoning of lemon, garlic, and parsley adds flavor without the need for heavy sauces or breading.

4. Broiling the tilapia keeps the cooking method healthy and avoids the extra calories and fat from frying

26. Turkey and Avocado Lettuce Wraps

Ingredient:

• 1 lb ground turkey
• 1 tsp olive oil
• 1 tsp chili powder
• 1/2 tsp cumin
• 1/4 tsp garlic powder
• Salt and pepper to taste
• 1 avocado, diced
• 1/4 cup diced red onion
• 2 tbsp chopped fresh cilantro
• 1 tbsp lime juice
• 8•10 large lettuce leaves (such as romaine or butter lettuce)

Instructions:

1. In a large skillet, cook the ground turkey over medium•high heat, breaking it up with a wooden spoon, until browned and cooked through, about 5•7 minutes.

2. Drain any excess fat from the skillet, then stir in the olive oil, chili powder, cumin, garlic powder, and a pinch of salt and pepper. Cook for 1 minute more.

3. In a small bowl, combine the diced avocado, red onion, cilantro, and lime juice. Season with a pinch of salt and pepper.

4. To assemble the wraps, place a couple of tablespoons of the seasoned turkey into the center of a lettuce leaf. Top with a spoonful of the avocado mixture.

5. Fold the sides of the lettuce leaf over the filling and enjoy.

These turkey and avocado lettuce wraps are an excellent choice for young men aiming for weight loss for several reasons:

1. Ground turkey is a lean protein that is lower in fat and calories compared to ground beef.

2. Avocado provides healthy fats, fiber, and nutrients to help keep you feeling full and satisfied.

3. The fresh lettuce leaves are a low•calorie, low•carb alternative to traditional bread or tortillas.

27. Mango and Black Bean Salad

Ingredient:

- 1 (15 oz) can black beans, rinsed and drained
- 1 ripe mango, diced
- 1 red bell pepper, diced
- 1 cup cherry tomatoes, halved
- 1/2 red onion, thinly sliced
- 1/4 cup chopped fresh cilantro
- 2 tbsp lime juice
- 1 tbsp olive oil
- 1 tsp honey
- 1/4 tsp ground cumin
- Salt and pepper to taste

Instructions:

1. In a large bowl, combine the rinsed and drained black beans, diced mango, diced bell pepper, cherry tomatoes, sliced red onion, and chopped cilantro.

2. In a small bowl, whisk together the lime juice, olive oil, honey, and ground cumin. Season with salt and pepper to taste.

3. Pour the dressing over the salad and toss gently to coat.

4. Refrigerate the salad for at least 30 minutes to allow the flavors to meld.

5. Serve chilled or at room temperature.

This mango and black bean salad is a refreshing and flavorful dish that is perfect for young men aiming for weight loss. The combination of sweet mango, savory black beans, and crunchy vegetables provides a balance of nutrients and textures. The lime•honey dressing adds a bright, tangy flavor that complements the other ingredients. This salad is low in calories, high in fiber, and packed with vitamins and minerals, making it a great choice for a healthy and satisfying meal or snack.

28. Stuffed Bell Peppers with Quinoa

Ingredient:

• 4 bell peppers (any color), halved and seeded
• 1 cup cooked quinoa
• 1 lb ground turkey or lean ground beef
• 1 onion, diced
• 3 cloves garlic, minced
• 1 can (15 oz) diced tomatoes
• 1 tsp dried oregano
• 1 tsp dried basil
• Salt and pepper to taste
• 1/2 cup shredded low•fat mozzarella cheese (optional)

Instructions:

1. Preheat the oven to 375°F.

2. In a large skillet, cook the ground turkey or beef over medium heat, breaking it up with a wooden spoon, until browned, about 5•7 minutes.

3. Add the onion and garlic to the skillet and cook for 2•3 minutes until fragrant.

4. Stir in the diced tomatoes, oregano, basil, salt, and pepper. Simmer for 5 minutes.

5. Remove the skillet from heat and stir in the cooked quinoa.

6. Stuff the quinoa and meat mixture into the hollowed•out bell pepper halves, packing it in tightly.

7. Place the stuffed bell peppers in a baking dish. If desired, top with the shredded mozzarella cheese.

8. Bake for 25•30 minutes, or until the peppers are tender and the filling is hot. Serve the stuffed bell peppers warm.

This dish is a great source of lean protein, complex carbohydrates, and fiber, making it a nutritious and filling meal for young men aiming for weight loss. The bell peppers provide a good source of vitamins and antioxidants, while the quinoa adds a boost of plant•based protein. Enjoy!

29. Grilled Salmon with Spinach Salad

Ingredient:

- 4 oz salmon fillet
- 2 cups fresh spinach leaves
- 1/2 cup cherry tomatoes, halved
- 1/4 cup sliced cucumber
- 1 tbsp olive oil
- 1 tbsp balsamic vinegar
- Salt and pepper to taste

Instructions:

1. Preheat grill or grill pan to medium·high heat.

2. Season the salmon fillet with salt and pepper.

3. Grill the salmon for 4·6 minutes per side, or until it flakes easily with a fork.

4. In a large bowl, combine the spinach, tomatoes, and cucumber.

5. Drizzle the olive oil and balsamic vinegar over the salad and toss to coat.

6. Serve the grilled salmon on top of the spinach salad.

This meal is high in protein from the salmon, and the spinach salad provides fiber, vitamins, and minerals. The healthy fats from the olive oil and the lean protein from the salmon make this a great option for young men aiming for weight loss. The portion size is also appropriate for weight management. Enjoy!

30. Hummus and Vegetable Platter

Ingredient:

• 1 cup homemade or store•bought hummus
• 1 cup baby carrots
• 1 cup cucumber slices
• 1 cup cherry tomatoes
• 1 cup bell pepper strips (red, yellow, or orange)
• 1 cup broccoli florets
• 1 cup cauliflower florets
• 1•2 tbsp olive oil (optional)
• Salt and pepper to taste

Instructions:

1. Arrange the vegetables on a large platter or plate, grouping them together for a visually appealing presentation.

2. Place the hummus in the center of the platter or in a small bowl.

3. If desired, drizzle a small amount of olive oil over the vegetables for added flavor and moisture.

4. Season the vegetables with a pinch of salt and pepper.

Serve the hummus and vegetable platter immediately, or cover and refrigerate until ready to serve.

This hummus and vegetable platter is a nutrient•dense, low•calorie option that is perfect for young men aiming for weight loss. The combination of protein•rich hummus and a variety of fresh, crunchy vegetables provides a satisfying and filling snack or light meal. The vegetables are high in fiber, vitamins, and minerals, while the hummus adds a creamy, flavorful dip that complements the veggies perfectly. This dish is a great way to incorporate more plant•based foods into your diet and support your weight loss goals.

31. Chicken and Avocado Salad

Ingredient:

• 2 cups cooked and shredded chicken breast
• 1 ripe avocado, diced
• 1 cup cherry tomatoes, halved
• 1/2 cup diced cucumber
• 1/4 cup diced red onion
• 2 tbsp chopped fresh cilantro
• 2 tbsp lime juice
• 1 tbsp olive oil
• 1 tsp Dijon mustard
• Salt and pepper to taste

Instructions:

1. In a large bowl, combine the shredded chicken, diced avocado, cherry tomatoes, diced cucumber, red onion, and chopped cilantro.

2. In a small bowl, whisk together the lime juice, olive oil, and Dijon mustard. Season with salt and pepper to taste.

3. Pour the dressing over the chicken and avocado salad and toss gently to coat.

4. Serve the salad immediately or refrigerate for up to 2 days.

This chicken and avocado salad is a great option for young men aiming for weight loss. It's packed with lean protein from the chicken, healthy fats from the avocado, and a variety of fresh vegetables. The lime•Dijon dressing adds a bright, tangy flavor that complements the other ingredients.

The combination of protein, healthy fats, and fiber from the vegetables and avocado will help keep you feeling full and satisfied, making this a great choice for a light lunch or dinner. Plus, it's easy to prepare and can be made ahead of time for a quick and nutritious meal.

32. Baked Tofu with Mixed Vegetables

Ingredient:

• 1 block (14 oz) extra•firm tofu, pressed and cubed
• 2 tbsp low•sodium soy sauce or tamari
• 1 tbsp sesame oil
• 1 tsp garlic powder
• 1 tsp ginger powder
• 1 cup broccoli florets
• 1 cup sliced mushrooms
• 1 cup sliced bell peppers
• 1 cup snow peas or snap peas
• 2 tbsp low•sodium vegetable broth
• 1 tbsp rice vinegar
• Salt and pepper to taste
• Chopped scallions for garnish (optional)

Instructions:

1. Preheat the oven to 400°F. Line a baking sheet with parchment paper.

2. In a bowl, toss the cubed tofu with the soy sauce, sesame oil, garlic powder, and ginger powder. Spread the tofu on the prepared baking sheet and bake for 20•25 minutes, flipping halfway, until golden brown.

3. In a large skillet or wok, heat the vegetable broth over medium•high heat. Add the broccoli, mushrooms, bell peppers, and snow peas. Sauté for 5•7 minutes, until the vegetables are tender•crisp.

4. Add the baked tofu and rice vinegar to the skillet. Toss everything together and season with salt and pepper to taste.

5. Serve the baked tofu and mixed vegetables hot, garnished with chopped scallions if desired.

This dish is packed with plant•based protein from the tofu, as well as a variety of nutrient•dense vegetables. The baking method for the tofu helps create a crispy texture without the need for frying. This meal is low in calories and high in fiber, making it a great option for young men aiming for weight loss.

33. Eggplant Parmesan (Baked)

Ingredient:

- 1 large eggplant, sliced into 1/2•inch thick rounds
- 1 cup whole wheat breadcrumbs
- 1/2 cup grated Parmesan cheese
- 2 tsp dried oregano
- 1 tsp garlic powder
- 1/4 tsp red pepper flakes (optional)
- 1 egg, beaten
- 1 cup marinara sauce
- 1 cup shredded part•skim mozzarella cheese

Instructions:

1. Preheat the oven to 375°F. Line a baking sheet with parchment paper.

2. In a shallow bowl, combine the breadcrumbs, Parmesan, oregano, garlic powder, and red pepper flakes (if using).

3. Dip the eggplant slices in the beaten egg, then coat them in the breadcrumb mixture, pressing gently to adhere.

4. Arrange the breaded eggplant slices in a single layer on the prepared baking sheet.

5. Bake for 20•25 minutes, flipping the slices halfway, until the eggplant is tender and the breading is golden brown.

6. Spread 1/2 cup of the marinara sauce in the bottom of a baking dish. Arrange the baked eggplant slices on top.

7. Sprinkle the mozzarella cheese over the eggplant.

8. Bake for an additional 10•15 minutes, or until the cheese is melted and bubbly.

9. Serve the baked eggplant parmesan warm, with the remaining marinara sauce on the side.

This baked eggplant parmesan dish is a healthier alternative to the traditional fried version, making it a great option for young men aiming for weight loss. The eggplant is a low•calorie, high•fiber vegetable, and the whole wheat breadcrumbs and reduced•fat cheese help keep the dish light and nutritious. Enjoy!

34. Chia Seed Pudding with Almond Milk

Ingredient:

• 1/4 cup chia seeds
• 1 cup unsweetened almond milk
• 1 tbsp honey or maple syrup (optional)
• 1 tsp vanilla extract
• 1/4 tsp ground cinnamon
• Fresh berries, sliced fruit, or nuts for topping (optional)

Instructions:

1. In a medium bowl, whisk together the chia seeds, almond milk, honey/maple syrup (if using), vanilla extract, and cinnamon until well combined.

2. Cover the bowl and refrigerate for at least 2 hours, or overnight, stirring occasionally, until the chia seeds have thickened the mixture into a pudding•like consistency.

3. Divide the chia seed pudding into individual serving bowls or jars.

4. Top the pudding with your choice of fresh berries, sliced fruit, or chopped nuts.

5. Serve chilled and enjoy!

This chia seed pudding is a nutritious and satisfying breakfast or snack option for young men aiming for weight loss. Chia seeds are packed with fiber, protein, and omega•3 fatty acids, which can help promote feelings of fullness and support overall health. The almond milk provides a creamy, dairy•free base, and the optional honey or maple syrup adds a touch of sweetness.

The fresh fruit and nuts on top provide additional nutrients, texture, and flavor. This recipe is easy to prepare in advance, making it a convenient and healthy choice for busy mornings or snack times. Enjoy this chia seed pudding as part of a balanced diet to support your weight loss goals.

35. Turkey Chili

Ingredient:

- 1 lb ground turkey breast
- 1 onion, diced
- 3 cloves garlic, minced
- 2 bell peppers, diced
- 2 cans (15 oz each) diced tomatoes
- 1 can (15 oz) kidney beans, rinsed and drained
- 2 tbsp chili powder
- 1 tsp cumin
- 1 tsp oregano
- 1/2 tsp cayenne pepper (optional, for spice)
- Salt and pepper to taste

Instructions:

1. In a large pot or Dutch oven, cook the ground turkey over medium·high heat, breaking it up with a wooden spoon, until browned, about 5·7 minutes.

2. Add the onion and garlic and cook for 2·3 minutes until fragrant.

3. Stir in the bell peppers, diced tomatoes, kidney beans, chili powder, cumin, oregano, and cayenne (if using). Season with salt and pepper.

4. Bring the chili to a simmer and let it cook for 20·25 minutes, stirring occasionally, until the flavors have melded and the chili has thickened.

5. Serve hot, garnished with chopped scallions, avocado, or a sprinkle of shredded cheese if desired.

This turkey chili is a great source of lean protein, fiber, and complex carbohydrates, making it a nutritious and filling meal for young men aiming for weight loss. The combination of spices adds lots of flavor without excessive calories or sodium. Enjoy!

36. Grilled Portobello Mushrooms

Ingredient:

• 4 large portobello mushroom caps, stems removed
• 2 tbsp olive oil
• 2 tbsp balsamic vinegar
• 2 cloves garlic, minced
• 1 tsp dried thyme
• Salt and pepper to taste
• Optional toppings: grilled vegetables, crumbled feta, balsamic glaze

Instructions:

1. Preheat your grill or grill pan to medium•high heat.

2. In a shallow dish, whisk together the olive oil, balsamic vinegar, minced garlic, and dried thyme.

3. Add the portobello mushroom caps to the dish and turn to coat both sides evenly with the marinade.

4. Grill the mushrooms for 4•5 minutes per side, or until they are tender and have grill marks.

5. Transfer the grilled portobello mushrooms to a serving plate and season with salt and pepper to taste.

6. If desired, top the grilled mushrooms with your choice of grilled vegetables, crumbled feta, or a drizzle of balsamic glaze.

7. Serve the grilled portobello mushrooms warm.

These grilled portobello mushrooms are a fantastic option for young men aiming for weight loss. Portobellos are a low•calorie, nutrient•dense vegetable that can provide a satisfying and filling meal. The grilling method adds a delicious, smoky flavor without the need for excessive oil or butter.

The balsamic marinade adds a tangy, savory element to the mushrooms, while the optional toppings can provide additional flavor and nutrients. Enjoy these grilled portobello mushrooms as a main dish, or serve them as a side to complement grilled or roasted proteins for a well•balanced and healthy meal.

37. Seared Scallops with Asparagus

Ingredient:

- 1 lb sea scallops, patted dry
- 1 tbsp olive oil
- 1 lb asparagus, trimmed and cut into 1•inch pieces
- 2 cloves garlic, minced
- 2 tbsp lemon juice
- 1 tbsp chopped fresh parsley
- Salt and pepper to taste

Instructions:

1. Heat a large skillet over high heat. Add the olive oil.

2. Season the scallops with salt and pepper. Working in batches if needed, sear the scallops for 2•3 minutes per side, until they develop a nice golden•brown crust. Transfer the seared scallops to a plate.

3. In the same skillet, add the asparagus and garlic. Sauté for 3•5 minutes, until the asparagus is tender•crisp.

4. Return the seared scallops to the skillet with the asparagus. Drizzle the lemon juice over the top and sprinkle with the chopped parsley.

5. Toss everything together gently and serve immediately.

This seared scallops with asparagus dish is a fantastic option for young men aiming for weight loss. Scallops are a lean, protein•rich seafood that is low in calories and high in nutrients. The asparagus provides fiber, vitamins, and minerals to create a well•balanced and nutrient•dense meal.

The quick searing method for the scallops helps to develop a delicious caramelized crust without the need for excessive oil or butter. The lemon juice and fresh parsley add bright, fresh flavors to the dish without adding unnecessary calories.

Enjoy this seared scallops with asparagus as a main course or as part of a larger balanced meal. It's a great way to incorporate healthy, lean protein and vegetables into your diet while supporting your weight loss goals.

38. Vegetable Soup

Ingredient:

• 1 tbsp olive oil
• 1 onion, diced
• 3 cloves garlic, minced
• 2 carrots, peeled and diced
• 2 celery stalks, diced
• 1 zucchini, diced
• 1 cup green beans, trimmed and cut into 1•inch pieces
• 1 (15 oz) can diced tomatoes
• 4 cups low•sodium vegetable or chicken broth
• 1 tsp dried thyme
• 1 tsp dried oregano
• Salt and pepper to taste
• 1 (15 oz) can kidney beans, rinsed and drained (optional)
• Chopped fresh parsley for garnish (optional)

Instructions:

1. In a large pot or Dutch oven, heat the olive oil over medium heat. Add the diced onion and sauté for 3•4 minutes until translucent.

2. Add the minced garlic and sauté for an additional minute until fragrant.

3. Stir in the diced carrots, celery, zucchini, and green beans. Sauté for 5•7 minutes, until the vegetables start to soften.

4. Pour in the diced tomatoes with their juices and the vegetable or chicken broth. Add the dried thyme and oregano, and season with salt and pepper to taste.

5. Bring the soup to a boil, then reduce the heat and let it simmer for 20•25 minutes, or until the vegetables are tender.

6. If using, stir in the rinsed and drained kidney beans and heat through. Ladle the vegetable soup into bowls and garnish with chopped fresh parsley, if desired.

This vegetable soup is a nutritious and filling option for young men aiming for weight loss. It's packed with a variety of fresh vegetables, providing a wealth of fiber, vitamins, and minerals. The broth•based soup is low in calories but high in flavor and satisfaction. The optional addition of kidney beans adds extra protein and fiber to make this a more substantial meal.

39. Grilled Swordfish with Mango Salsa

Ingredient:

For the Mango Salsa:
• 1 ripe mango, diced
• 1/2 red onion, finely chopped
• 1 jalapeño, seeded and finely chopped
• 1/4 cup chopped fresh cilantro
• 2 tbsp lime juice
• 1 tsp olive oil
• Salt and pepper to taste

For the Swordfish:
• 4 (6 oz) swordfish steaks
• 1 tbsp olive oil
• 1 tsp chili powder
• 1 tsp garlic powder
• Salt and pepper to taste

Instructions:

1. Make the mango salsa: In a medium bowl, combine the diced mango, chopped red onion, jalapeño, cilantro, lime juice, and olive oil. Season with salt and pepper to taste. Cover and refrigerate until ready to serve.

2. Prepare the swordfish: Preheat your grill or grill pan to medium•high heat.

3. Brush the swordfish steaks with the olive oil and season both sides with the chili powder, garlic powder, salt, and pepper.

4. Grill the swordfish for 4•5 minutes per side, or until it flakes easily with a fork and is cooked through.

5. Serve the grilled swordfish steaks topped with the chilled mango salsa.

This grilled swordfish with mango salsa is a light, flavorful, and nutrient•dense meal that is perfect for young men aiming for weight loss. The swordfish provides a lean source of protein, while the mango salsa adds a refreshing, sweet•and•spicy contrast. The combination of the grilled fish and the vibrant salsa makes for a delicious and visually appealing dish.

40. Cucumber and Tomato Salad

Ingredient:

- 2 cups diced cucumber
- 1 cup halved cherry or grape tomatoes
- 1/4 cup diced red onion
- 2 tbsp chopped fresh basil
- 1 tbsp olive oil
- 1 tbsp red wine vinegar
- 1 tsp Dijon mustard
- 1 tsp honey
- Salt and pepper to taste

Instructions:

1. In a large bowl, combine the diced cucumber, halved tomatoes, and diced red onion.

2. In a small bowl, whisk together the olive oil, red wine vinegar, Dijon mustard, and honey. Season with salt and pepper to taste.

3. Pour the dressing over the cucumber and tomato mixture and toss gently to coat.

4. Sprinkle the chopped fresh basil over the salad and toss again.

5. Refrigerate the salad for at least 30 minutes to allow the flavors to meld.

6. Serve chilled or at room temperature.

This cucumber and tomato salad is a refreshing and nutritious option for young men aiming for weight loss. The combination of crisp cucumbers, juicy tomatoes, and tangy red onion provides a variety of textures and flavors. The simple dressing of olive oil, vinegar, mustard, and honey adds a light, flavorful coating without adding excessive calories or fat.

The fresh basil adds a bright, herbal note that complements the other ingredients. This salad is low in calories but high in fiber, vitamins, and antioxidants, making it a great choice for a light lunch or side dish. The hydrating properties of the cucumbers and the nutrient•dense tomatoes also make this salad a healthy and satisfying option for supporting your weight loss goals.

41. Chicken and Quinoa Bowls

Ingredient:

- 1 cup uncooked quinoa, rinsed
- 2 cups low•sodium chicken broth
- 1 lb boneless, skinless chicken breasts
- 1 tsp olive oil
- 1 tsp garlic powder
- 1 tsp dried oregano
- Salt and pepper to taste
- 1 cup diced cucumber
- 1 cup cherry tomatoes, halved
- 1/2 cup diced red onion
- 1/4 cup crumbled feta cheese (optional)
- 2 tbsp chopped fresh parsley
- 2 tbsp lemon juice

Instructions:

1. In a medium saucepan, combine the rinsed quinoa and chicken broth. Bring to a boil, then reduce heat, cover, and simmer for 15•20 minutes, until the quinoa is tender and the liquid is absorbed. Fluff with a fork and set aside.

2. Preheat the oven to 400°F. Season the chicken breasts with the garlic powder, oregano, salt, and pepper.

3. Heat the olive oil in a large oven•safe skillet over medium•high heat. Add the chicken and sear for 2•3 minutes per side to get a nice golden•brown crust.

4. Transfer the skillet to the preheated oven and bake for 12•15 minutes, or until the chicken is cooked through and reaches an internal temperature of 165°F. Allow the chicken to rest for 5 minutes, then slice or shred it.

5. In a large bowl, combine the cooked quinoa, sliced or shredded chicken, diced cucumber, cherry tomatoes, red onion, feta cheese (if using), and chopped parsley.

6. Drizzle the lemon juice over the bowl and toss gently to combine. Serve the chicken and quinoa bowls warm or chilled.

This chicken and quinoa bowl is a nutritious and filling meal that is perfect for young men aiming for weight loss. The combination of lean protein from the chicken, complex carbohydrates from the quinoa, and a variety of fresh vegetables provides a balanced and satisfying dish. Enjoy!

42. Roasted Cauliflower with Turmeric

Ingredient:

• 1 head of cauliflower, cut into florets
• 2 tbsp olive oil
• 1 tsp ground turmeric
• 1 tsp ground cumin
• 1/2 tsp garlic powder
• 1/4 tsp cayenne pepper (optional, for a spicy kick)
• Salt and pepper to taste
• Chopped fresh parsley for garnish (optional)

Instructions:

1. Preheat your oven to 400°F. Line a large baking sheet with parchment paper.

2. In a large bowl, toss the cauliflower florets with the olive oil, turmeric, cumin, garlic powder, and cayenne pepper (if using). Season with salt and pepper.

3. Spread the seasoned cauliflower in a single layer on the prepared baking sheet.

4. Roast the cauliflower for 20•25 minutes, flipping halfway, until it's tender and lightly browned.

5. Remove the roasted cauliflower from the oven and transfer it to a serving dish.

6. Garnish the roasted cauliflower with chopped fresh parsley, if desired.

7. Serve the turmeric•roasted cauliflower warm.

This roasted cauliflower with turmeric is a delicious and nutritious side dish that's perfect for young men aiming for weight loss. Cauliflower is a low•calorie, high•fiber vegetable that's packed with vitamins, minerals, and antioxidants. The addition of turmeric, cumin, and garlic powder adds a flavorful, aromatic seasoning to the cauliflower without the need for excessive salt or unhealthy fats.

The roasting method brings out the natural sweetness of the cauliflower and creates a crispy, caramelized exterior. This dish is a great way to incorporate more nutrient•dense vegetables into your diet while supporting your weight loss goals. Enjoy the roasted cauliflower on its own or as a side to grilled or baked proteins for a well•balanced and satisfying meal.

43. Spicy Black Bean Soup

Ingredient:

• 1 tbsp olive oil
• 1 onion, diced
• 3 cloves garlic, minced
• 2 tsp ground cumin
• 1 tsp chili powder
• 1/4 tsp cayenne pepper (or to taste)
• 2 (15 oz) cans black beans, rinsed and drained
• 4 cups low•sodium vegetable or chicken broth
• 1 (14.5 oz) can diced tomatoes
• 1 bay leaf
• Salt and pepper to taste
• Chopped fresh cilantro for garnish (optional)
• Lime wedges for serving (optional)

Instructions:

1. In a large pot or Dutch oven, heat the olive oil over medium heat. Add the diced onion and sauté for 3•4 minutes until translucent.

2. Add the minced garlic, ground cumin, chili powder, and cayenne pepper. Sauté for 1 minute, until fragrant.

3. Stir in the rinsed and drained black beans, vegetable or chicken broth, diced tomatoes, and bay leaf. Season with salt and pepper to taste.

4. Bring the soup to a boil, then reduce the heat and let it simmer for 20•25 minutes, stirring occasionally, until the flavors have melded and the soup has thickened slightly.

5. Remove the bay leaf. Using an immersion blender or regular blender, puree about half of the soup to create a creamy texture, leaving the other half chunky.

6. Ladle the spicy black bean soup into bowls and garnish with chopped fresh cilantro, if desired. Serve the soup with lime wedges on the side.

This spicy black bean soup is a nutritious and flavorful option for young men aiming for weight loss. Black beans are a great source of plant•based protein, fiber, and complex carbohydrates, making this soup a filling and satisfying meal. The blend of spices adds a delicious kick of heat without excessive calories or sodium.

44. Baked Sweet Potato Fries

Ingredient:

• 2 medium sweet potatoes, peeled and cut into 1/2•inch thick fries
• 1 tbsp olive oil
• 1 tsp paprika
• 1/2 tsp garlic powder
• 1/2 tsp onion powder
• 1/4 tsp cayenne pepper (optional, for a spicy kick)
• Salt and pepper to taste

Instructions:

1. Preheat the oven to 400°F. Line a baking sheet with parchment paper.

2. In a large bowl, toss the sweet potato fries with the olive oil, paprika, garlic powder, onion powder, and cayenne pepper (if using). Season with salt and pepper.

3. Spread the seasoned sweet potato fries in a single layer on the prepared baking sheet.

4. Bake for 20•25 minutes, flipping the fries halfway, until they are tender and lightly browned.

5. Serve the baked sweet potato fries hot, seasoning with additional salt and pepper if desired.

These baked sweet potato fries are a healthier alternative to traditional french fries, making them a great option for young men aiming for weight loss. Sweet potatoes are a nutrient•dense carbohydrate source, providing fiber, vitamins, and minerals. The baking method avoids the extra calories and fat from frying, while the spices add flavor without the need for excessive salt or unhealthy toppings.

Enjoy these baked sweet potato fries as a side dish or a satisfying snack. They pair well with grilled or baked proteins, such as chicken or fish, for a balanced and nutritious meal. The combination of complex carbohydrates, fiber, and healthy fats can help keep you feeling full and satisfied, supporting your weight loss goals.

45. Chicken Lettuce Wraps

Ingredient:

- 1 lb ground or finely chopped chicken breast
- 1 tbsp sesame oil
- 2 cloves garlic, minced
- 1 tbsp grated fresh ginger
- 2 tbsp low•sodium soy sauce
- 1 tbsp rice vinegar
- 1 tsp honey
- 1/4 tsp red pepper flakes (optional)
- 1 cup shredded carrots
- 1 cup thinly sliced mushrooms
- 1/2 cup diced water chestnuts
- 1/4 cup chopped green onions
- 12•16 large lettuce leaves (such as romaine, bibb, or butter lettuce)

Instructions:

1. In a large skillet or wok, heat the sesame oil over medium•high heat. Add the ground or chopped chicken and cook, breaking it up with a wooden spoon, until no longer pink, about 5•7 minutes.

2. Add the minced garlic and grated ginger to the skillet and cook for 1 minute, until fragrant.

3. Stir in the soy sauce, rice vinegar, honey, and red pepper flakes (if using). Cook for 2•3 minutes, until the sauce has thickened slightly.

4. Add the shredded carrots, sliced mushrooms, diced water chestnuts, and chopped green onions to the skillet. Toss everything together and cook for an additional 2•3 minutes.

5. To serve, spoon the chicken mixture into the lettuce leaves. Wrap the lettuce around the filling and enjoy.

These chicken lettuce wraps are a fantastic option for young men aiming for weight loss. The lean ground chicken provides a good source of protein, while the fresh vegetables and crunchy water chestnuts add fiber, vitamins, and minerals. The flavorful sauce made with soy sauce, rice vinegar, and honey adds a delicious Asian•inspired taste without excessive calories or sodium.

The lettuce leaves act as a low•calorie, nutrient•dense wrapper, making this dish a great way to enjoy a satisfying meal without the heavy carbs of traditional wraps or buns. Enjoy these chicken lettuce wraps as a light lunch or dinner, or serve them as a healthy appetizer.

46. Grilled Mahi•Mahi with Veggies

Ingredient:

- 4 (6 oz) mahi•mahi fillets
- 2 tbsp olive oil, divided
- 1 tsp lemon zest
- 1 tbsp lemon juice
- 1 tsp dried oregano
- Salt and pepper to taste
- 1 zucchini, sliced into rounds
- 1 yellow squash, sliced into rounds
- 1 red bell pepper, sliced
- 1 red onion, sliced
- 2 cloves garlic, minced
- 1 tbsp chopped fresh parsley

Instructions:

1. Preheat your grill or grill pan to medium•high heat.

2. In a shallow dish, combine 1 tbsp of the olive oil, lemon zest, lemon juice, dried oregano, and a pinch of salt and pepper. Add the mahi•mahi fillets and turn to coat both sides.

3. In a large bowl, toss the sliced zucchini, yellow squash, bell pepper, and red onion with the remaining 1 tbsp of olive oil, minced garlic, and a pinch of salt and pepper.

4. Grill the mahi•mahi fillets for 4•5 minutes per side, or until the fish flakes easily with a fork.

5. Grill the vegetable mixture for 5•7 minutes, stirring occasionally, until the vegetables are tender•crisp.

6. Transfer the grilled mahi•mahi and vegetables to a serving platter. Sprinkle the chopped fresh parsley over the top. Serve the grilled mahi•mahi and vegetables immediately.

This grilled mahi•mahi with vegetables is a fantastic option for young men aiming for weight loss. Mahi•mahi is a lean, flavorful fish that is high in protein and low in calories. The combination of grilled vegetables provides a variety of nutrients, fiber, and antioxidants.

The simple lemon•oregano marinade for the fish and the minimal oil used for the vegetables keep this dish light and healthy. The grilling method adds a delicious smoky flavor without the need for excessive fats or sauces.

47. Spicy Kale Chips

Ingredient:

- 1 bunch kale, stems removed and leaves torn into bite•sized pieces
- 1 tbsp olive oil
- 1 tsp chili powder
- 1/2 tsp garlic powder
- 1/4 tsp cayenne pepper (or to taste)
- 1/4 tsp salt

Instructions:

1. Preheat your oven to 350°F. Line a large baking sheet with parchment paper.

2. In a large bowl, toss the kale leaves with the olive oil, chili powder, garlic powder, cayenne pepper, and salt until the kale is evenly coated.

3. Spread the kale leaves in a single layer on the prepared baking sheet, making sure they are not overlapping.

4. Bake for 12•15 minutes, flipping the kale halfway, until the leaves are crispy and lightly browned.

5. Remove the spicy kale chips from the oven and let them cool for a few minutes before serving.

These spicy kale chips are a fantastic snack option for young men aiming for weight loss. Kale is a nutrient•dense, low•calorie green that is packed with fiber, vitamins, and antioxidants. The combination of chili powder, garlic powder, and cayenne pepper adds a delicious spicy kick without excessive calories or sodium.

The baking method helps to create a crispy, chip•like texture without the need for frying in oil. This makes the kale chips a much healthier alternative to traditional potato or tortilla chips.

Enjoy these spicy kale chips as a satisfying and nutritious snack throughout the day. The fiber and nutrients in the kale can help keep you feeling full and satisfied, supporting your weight loss goals. You can also experiment with different seasoning blends to keep the snack interesting and flavorful.

48. Turkey and Veggie Stir•Fry

Ingredient:

- 1 lb ground turkey
- 2 tbsp low•sodium soy sauce
- 1 tbsp rice vinegar
- 1 tsp sesame oil
- 1 tsp cornstarch
- 2 tsp olive oil
- 3 cloves garlic, minced
- 1 tbsp grated fresh ginger
- 1 red bell pepper, sliced
- 1 cup broccoli florets
- 1 cup sliced mushrooms
- 1 cup snow peas or snap peas
- 2 green onions, sliced
- Salt and pepper to taste
- Chopped cilantro for garnish (optional)

Instructions:

1. In a medium bowl, combine the ground turkey, soy sauce, rice vinegar, sesame oil, and cornstarch. Mix well and set aside.

2. Heat the olive oil in a large skillet or wok over high heat. Add the minced garlic and grated ginger and cook for 1 minute, until fragrant.

3. Add the marinated ground turkey to the skillet and cook, breaking it up with a wooden spoon, for 3•4 minutes, until no longer pink.

4. Add the sliced bell pepper, broccoli florets, mushrooms, and snow peas or snap peas to the skillet. Stir•fry for 4•5 minutes, until the vegetables are tender•crisp.

5. Stir in the sliced green onions and season with salt and pepper to taste.

6. Serve the turkey and veggie stir•fry hot, garnished with chopped cilantro if desired.

This turkey and veggie stir•fry is a fantastic option for young men aiming for weight loss. Ground turkey is a lean protein source that is low in calories and high in nutrients. The combination of fresh vegetables provides a variety of fiber, vitamins, and minerals.

The quick stir•fry cooking method helps to preserve the nutrients in the vegetables and keeps the dish light and flavorful. The simple sauce made with soy sauce, rice vinegar, and sesame oil adds a delicious Asian•inspired taste without excessive calories or sodium.

49. Carrot and Ginger Soup

Ingredient:

• 1 lb carrots, peeled and chopped
• 1 onion, diced
• 3 cloves garlic, minced
• 1 tbsp grated fresh ginger
• 4 cups low•sodium vegetable or chicken broth
• 1 cup unsweetened almond milk
• 1 tsp ground cumin
• 1/4 tsp cayenne pepper (optional)
• Salt and pepper to taste
• Chopped fresh cilantro or parsley for garnish (optional)

Instructions:

1. In a large pot or Dutch oven, heat a drizzle of olive oil over medium heat. Add the chopped carrots, diced onion, minced garlic, and grated ginger. Sauté for 5•7 minutes, stirring occasionally, until the vegetables are softened.

2. Pour in the vegetable or chicken broth and bring the mixture to a boil. Reduce the heat and let the soup simmer for 15•20 minutes, or until the carrots are very tender.

3. Using an immersion blender or a regular blender, puree the soup until smooth and creamy.

4. Stir in the unsweetened almond milk, ground cumin, and cayenne pepper (if using). Season with salt and pepper to taste.

5. Reheat the soup if necessary, then serve hot, garnished with chopped fresh cilantro or parsley, if desired.

This carrot and ginger soup is a nourishing and flavorful option for young men aiming for weight loss. The carrots provide a good source of beta•carotene and fiber, while the ginger adds a warm, slightly spicy kick. The almond milk makes the soup creamy without adding excessive calories or fat. This soup is low in calories but high in nutrients, making it a satisfying and healthy choice for a light meal or snack.

50. Zucchini Fritters

Ingredient:

• 2 medium zucchini, grated
• 1 egg, lightly beaten
• 2 tbsp whole wheat flour
• 2 tbsp grated Parmesan cheese
• 2 tbsp chopped fresh parsley
• 1 clove garlic, minced
• 1/4 tsp baking powder
• Salt and pepper to taste
• 1 tbsp olive oil

Instructions:

1. Grate the zucchini using a box grater or food processor. Place the grated zucchini in a clean kitchen towel or cheesecloth and squeeze out as much moisture as possible.

2. In a medium bowl, combine the grated zucchini, beaten egg, whole wheat flour, Parmesan cheese, chopped parsley, minced garlic, and baking powder. Season with salt and pepper.

3. Heat the olive oil in a large non•stick skillet over medium heat.

4. Scoop heaping tablespoons of the zucchini mixture and gently place them in the hot skillet, flattening them slightly with a spatula to form fritters.

5. Cook the zucchini fritters for 2•3 minutes per side, or until golden brown.

6. Transfer the cooked fritters to a paper towel•lined plate to drain any excess oil.

7. Serve the zucchini fritters warm, garnished with additional chopped parsley if desired.

These zucchini fritters are a fantastic option for young men aiming for weight loss. Zucchini is a low•calorie, high•fiber vegetable that provides a good source of vitamins and minerals. The addition of whole wheat flour, Parmesan cheese, and egg helps to bind the fritters and add a boost of protein.

The pan•frying method uses a minimal amount of olive oil, keeping the fritters light and crispy without excessive fat or calories. Enjoy these zucchini fritters as a side dish or a light main course, paired with a fresh salad or roasted vegetables for a complete and nutritious meal.

51. Avocado and Tomato Salad

Ingredient:

- 2 ripe avocados, diced
- 1 pint cherry or grape tomatoes, halved
- 1/2 red onion, thinly sliced
- 1/4 cup fresh basil leaves, chopped
- 2 tbsp olive oil
- 2 tbsp balsamic vinegar
- 1 tsp Dijon mustard
- 1 tsp honey
- Salt and pepper to taste

Instructions:

1. In a large bowl, gently combine the diced avocado, halved tomatoes, and sliced red onion.

2. In a small bowl, whisk together the olive oil, balsamic vinegar, Dijon mustard, and honey. Season with salt and pepper to taste.

3. Pour the dressing over the avocado and tomato mixture and toss gently to coat.

4. Sprinkle the chopped fresh basil over the salad and toss again.

5. Serve the avocado and tomato salad immediately, or refrigerate for up to 30 minutes before serving.

This avocado and tomato salad is a refreshing and nutrient·dense option for young men aiming for weight loss. The combination of creamy avocado, juicy tomatoes, and tangy red onion provides a variety of flavors and textures.

The simple dressing made with olive oil, balsamic vinegar, Dijon, and honey adds a light, flavorful coating without excessive calories or fat. The fresh basil provides a bright, herbal note that complements the other ingredients.

This salad is low in calories but high in healthy fats from the avocado, as well as fiber, vitamins, and antioxidants from the tomatoes and other vegetables. The hydrating properties of the salad also make it a great choice for supporting your weight loss goals.

Enjoy this avocado and tomato salad as a light lunch or side dish, or pair it with grilled or baked proteins for a complete and balanced meal.

52. Grilled Vegetable Kabobs

Ingredient:

- 1 zucchini, cut into 1•inch chunks
- 1 yellow squash, cut into 1•inch chunks
- 1 red bell pepper, cut into 1•inch pieces
- 1 red onion, cut into 1•inch pieces
- 8 oz cremini or button mushrooms, halved
- 2 tbsp olive oil
- 1 tsp dried oregano
- 1 tsp garlic powder
- Salt and pepper to taste
- Wooden or metal skewers

Instructions:

1. Preheat your grill or grill pan to medium•high heat.

2. In a large bowl, toss the chopped zucchini, yellow squash, bell pepper, onion, and mushrooms with the olive oil, dried oregano, garlic powder, salt, and pepper until evenly coated.

3. Thread the vegetables onto the skewers, alternating the different types of vegetables.

4. Grill the vegetable kabobs for 12•15 minutes, turning occasionally, until the vegetables are tender and lightly charred. Serve the grilled vegetable kabobs hot.

These grilled vegetable kabobs are a fantastic option for young men aiming for weight loss. The combination of fresh, colorful vegetables provides a variety of nutrients, fiber, and antioxidants. The grilling method adds a delicious smoky flavor without the need for excessive oils or sauces.

The simple seasoning of olive oil, oregano, and garlic powder enhances the natural flavors of the vegetables without adding unnecessary calories or sodium. The kabob format makes this dish easy to prepare and serve, and the variety of vegetables ensures a well•balanced and satisfying meal.

Enjoy the grilled vegetable kabobs as a main dish or as a side to grilled or baked proteins. The fiber and nutrients in the vegetables can help keep you feeling full and satisfied, supporting your weight loss goals.

53. Chicken and Broccoli Stir•Fry

Ingredient:

• 1 lb boneless, skinless chicken breasts, cut into 1•inch pieces
• 2 tbsp low•sodium soy sauce
• 1 tbsp rice vinegar
• 1 tsp sesame oil
• 1 tsp cornstarch
• 2 tsp olive oil
• 3 cloves garlic, minced
• 1 tbsp grated fresh ginger
• 4 cups broccoli florets
• 1/4 cup low•sodium chicken or vegetable broth
• 1 tsp honey
• Salt and pepper to taste
• Chopped green onions and sesame seeds for garnish (optional)

Instructions:

1. In a medium bowl, combine the cubed chicken, soy sauce, rice vinegar, sesame oil, and cornstarch. Toss to coat the chicken and set aside.

2. Heat the olive oil in a large skillet or wok over high heat. Add the minced garlic and grated ginger and cook for 1 minute, until fragrant.

3. Add the marinated chicken to the skillet and stir•fry for 3•4 minutes, until the chicken is mostly cooked through.

4. Add the broccoli florets and the chicken broth to the skillet. Cover and cook for 3•4 minutes, until the broccoli is tender•crisp.

5. Uncover the skillet and stir in the honey. Season with salt and pepper to taste.

6. Continue to stir•fry the chicken and broccoli for an additional 2•3 minutes, until the sauce has thickened slightly. Serve the chicken and broccoli stir•fry hot, garnished with chopped green onions and sesame seeds, if desired.

This chicken and broccoli stir•fry is a healthy and flavorful option for young men aiming for weight loss. The lean chicken provides a good source of protein, while the broccoli adds fiber, vitamins, and minerals. The simple sauce made with soy sauce, rice vinegar, and honey adds a delicious Asian•inspired flavor without excessive calories or sodium.

54. Pumpkin Soup

Ingredient:

- 1 (15 oz) can pumpkin puree
- 4 cups low·sodium vegetable or chicken broth
- 1 onion, diced
- 2 cloves garlic, minced
- 1 tsp ground cumin
- 1/2 tsp ground cinnamon
- 1/4 tsp ground nutmeg
- 1/4 tsp cayenne pepper (optional)
- Salt and black pepper to taste
- 2 tbsp plain Greek yogurt (for serving, optional)
- Chopped fresh parsley or chives for garnish (optional)

Instructions:

1. In a large pot or Dutch oven, sauté the onion in a small amount of olive oil or broth over medium heat for 3·4 minutes until translucent.

2. Add the garlic and sauté for 1 minute more until fragrant.

3. Stir in the pumpkin puree, broth, cumin, cinnamon, nutmeg, and cayenne (if using). Season with salt and pepper to taste.

4. Bring the soup to a simmer and let it cook for 10·15 minutes, stirring occasionally, until heated through.

5. Carefully transfer the soup to a blender and blend until smooth and creamy. You can also use an immersion blender right in the pot.

6. Serve the pumpkin soup warm, topped with a dollop of Greek yogurt and garnished with fresh parsley or chives, if desired.

This pumpkin soup is low in calories and fat, but high in fiber, vitamins, and antioxidants from the pumpkin. It makes a great starter or light main dish. Enjoy!

55. Lentil and Veggie Stew

Ingredient:

- 1 cup dry brown or green lentils, rinsed
- 4 cups low•sodium vegetable broth
- 1 tbsp olive oil
- 1 onion, diced
- 3 cloves garlic, minced
- 2 carrots, peeled and diced
- 2 celery stalks, diced
- 1 zucchini, diced
- 1 (14.5 oz) can diced tomatoes
- 2 tsp dried thyme
- 1 tsp dried oregano
- 1/4 tsp cayenne pepper (optional)
- Salt and black pepper to taste
- Fresh parsley for garnish (optional)

Instructions:

1. In a large pot, combine the lentils and vegetable broth. Bring to a boil, then reduce heat and simmer for 15•20 minutes, until lentils are tender.

2. In a separate large pot or Dutch oven, heat the olive oil over medium heat. Add the onion and sauté for 3•4 minutes until translucent.

3. Add the garlic, carrots, celery, and zucchini. Sauté for 5•7 minutes, stirring occasionally, until vegetables start to soften.

4. Stir in the cooked lentils, diced tomatoes, thyme, oregano, and cayenne (if using). Season with salt and pepper to taste.

5. Bring the stew to a simmer and let it cook for 10•15 minutes, allowing the flavors to meld.

6. Serve the lentil and veggie stew hot, garnished with fresh parsley if desired.

This hearty stew is packed with fiber, protein, and nutrients from the lentils and vegetables. It's low in calories and fat, making it an excellent choice for young men aiming to lose weight. Enjoy!

56. Baked Eggplant Slices

Ingredient:

• 1 large eggplant, sliced into 1/2•inch thick rounds
• 2 tbsp olive oil
• 1 tsp garlic powder
• 1 tsp dried oregano
• 1/4 tsp salt
• 1/4 tsp black pepper
• 1/2 cup grated Parmesan cheese (optional)

Instructions:

1. Preheat oven to 400°F. Line a baking sheet with parchment paper.

2. In a shallow bowl, combine the olive oil, garlic powder, oregano, salt, and pepper. Dip the eggplant slices into the oil mixture, coating both sides.

3. Arrange the eggplant slices in a single layer on the prepared baking sheet.

4. Bake for 15•20 minutes, flipping the slices halfway through, until the eggplant is tender and lightly browned.

5. If using Parmesan cheese, sprinkle it over the baked eggplant slices and return to the oven for 2•3 minutes until the cheese is melted.

6. Serve the baked eggplant slices warm. They can be enjoyed as a side dish or as a healthy snack.

This recipe is low in calories and carbs, making it a great option for young men aiming for weight loss. The eggplant provides fiber and nutrients, while the baking method avoids the extra calories from frying. Enjoy!

57. Shrimp and Avocado Salad

Ingredient:

- 1 lb cooked shrimp, peeled and deveined
- 2 avocados, diced
- 1 cup cherry tomatoes, halved
- 1/2 red onion, thinly sliced
- 1 tbsp olive oil
- 2 tbsp fresh lime juice
- 1 tbsp chopped fresh cilantro
- Salt and black pepper to taste

Instructions:

1. In a large bowl, gently combine the cooked shrimp, diced avocado, cherry tomatoes, and red onion slices.

2. In a small bowl, whisk together the olive oil, lime juice, and chopped cilantro. Season with salt and pepper.

3. Pour the dressing over the shrimp and avocado mixture and toss gently to coat.

4. Serve the shrimp and avocado salad chilled or at room temperature. It can be enjoyed on its own or over a bed of mixed greens.

This salad is an excellent choice for young men aiming for weight loss for a few reasons:

- Shrimp is a lean protein that is low in calories and fat, but high in nutrients.
- Avocado provides healthy fats, fiber, and nutrients to help keep you feeling full.
- The fresh vegetables add volume and antioxidants without a lot of calories.
- The simple dressing is light and flavorful without weighing down the dish.

This salad makes for a satisfying and nutritious meal or snack that can support weight loss goals. Enjoy!

58. Spinach and Feta Stuffed Chicken

Ingredient:

- 4 boneless, skinless chicken breasts
- 2 cups fresh spinach, chopped
- 1/2 cup crumbled feta cheese
- 2 cloves garlic, minced
- 1 tbsp olive oil
- Salt and pepper to taste

Instructions:

1. Preheat your oven to 400°F. Lightly grease a baking dish or line a baking sheet with parchment paper.

2. Slice each chicken breast horizontally to create a pocket, being careful not to cut all the way through.

3. In a medium bowl, combine the chopped spinach, crumbled feta, and minced garlic. Season with a pinch of salt and pepper.

4. Stuff the spinach and feta mixture evenly into the pockets of the chicken breasts.

5. Place the stuffed chicken breasts in the prepared baking dish or on the baking sheet. Drizzle the top of each chicken breast with a small amount of olive oil.

6. Bake the stuffed chicken for 25·30 minutes, or until the chicken is cooked through and the internal temperature reaches 165°F. Serve the spinach and feta stuffed chicken warm.

This spinach and feta stuffed chicken is a delicious and nutritious option for young men aiming for weight loss. The lean chicken breast provides a good source of protein, while the spinach and feta filling adds flavor, fiber, and healthy fats.

The baking method helps keep the chicken moist and juicy without the need for excessive oil or butter. This dish is low in calories but high in nutrients, making it a great choice for a balanced and satisfying meal.

Serve the spinach and feta stuffed chicken with a side of roasted vegetables or a fresh salad for a complete and healthy dinner. The combination of lean protein, vegetables, and healthy fats will help keep you feeling full and satisfied, supporting your weight loss goals.

59. Roasted Butternut Squash

Ingredient:

• 1 medium butternut squash, peeled, seeded, and cut into 1•inch cubes (about 4 cups)
• 2 tbsp olive oil
• 1 tsp ground cinnamon
• 1/2 tsp ground cumin
• 1/4 tsp ground nutmeg
• 1/4 tsp salt
• 1/4 tsp black pepper
• 2 tbsp chopped fresh parsley (optional)

Instructions:

1. Preheat your oven to 400°F (200°C). Line a large baking sheet with parchment paper.

2. In a large bowl, toss the cubed butternut squash with the olive oil, cinnamon, cumin, nutmeg, salt, and black pepper until the squash is evenly coated.

3. Spread the seasoned squash cubes in a single layer on the prepared baking sheet.

4. Roast the squash for 25•30 minutes, flipping the pieces halfway through, until the squash is tender and lightly browned.

5. Remove the roasted butternut squash from the oven and transfer to a serving dish.

6. If desired, sprinkle the roasted squash with the chopped fresh parsley before serving.

This roasted butternut squash makes a delicious and nutritious side dish or can be enjoyed as a healthy snack. The combination of warm spices complements the natural sweetness of the squash perfectly.

Butternut squash is an excellent source of vitamins A and C, as well as fiber and complex carbohydrates. It's a great option for those looking to incorporate more nutrient•dense vegetables into their diet.

Enjoy this simple yet flavorful roasted butternut squash recipe!

60. Cauliflower Tacos

Ingredient:

- 1 head of cauliflower, cut into small florets
- 2 tbsp olive oil
- 1 tsp chili powder
- 1 tsp cumin
- 1/2 tsp garlic powder
- 1/4 tsp salt
- 8•10 small corn or flour tortillas
- 1 cup shredded cabbage or lettuce
- 1 avocado, sliced
- 1/4 cup crumbled feta or queso fresco
- Chopped cilantro for garnish
- Lime wedges for serving

Instructions:

1. Preheat your oven to 400°F (200°C). Line a baking sheet with parchment paper.

2. In a large bowl, toss the cauliflower florets with the olive oil, chili powder, cumin, garlic powder, and salt until evenly coated.

3. Spread the seasoned cauliflower in a single layer on the prepared baking sheet.

4. Roast the cauliflower for 20•25 minutes, stirring halfway, until it's tender and lightly browned.

5. Warm the tortillas according to package instructions.

6. To assemble the tacos, place a few pieces of roasted cauliflower in each tortilla. Top with shredded cabbage or lettuce, sliced avocado, crumbled feta or queso fresco, and chopped cilantro.

7. Serve the cauliflower tacos immediately with lime wedges on the side.

These cauliflower tacos are a delicious and healthy vegetarian option. The roasted cauliflower provides a meaty texture and the spices add great flavor. The fresh toppings and tangy lime juice balance the dish perfectly.

Cauliflower is a nutrient•dense vegetable that's low in calories but high in fiber, vitamins, and minerals. It's a great alternative to meat in tacos, making this a great option for those looking to incorporate more plant•based meals into their diet.

61. Mushroom and Spinach Omelette

Ingredient:

- 3 large eggs
- 1 tbsp milk or water
- 1 tsp olive oil
- 1/2 cup sliced mushrooms
- 1 cup fresh spinach leaves
- 1 tbsp grated Parmesan cheese (optional)
- Salt and black pepper to taste

Instructions:

1. In a small bowl, whisk together the eggs and milk/water. Season with a pinch of salt and pepper.

2. Heat the olive oil in a small non•stick skillet over medium heat.

3. Add the sliced mushrooms and sauté for 2•3 minutes until softened.

4. Add the fresh spinach leaves and cook for 1 minute, stirring, until the spinach is wilted.

5. Pour the egg mixture into the skillet. As the eggs start to set around the edges, use a spatula to gently push the cooked edges towards the center, tilting the pan to allow the uncooked egg to flow to the edges.

6. When the eggs are mostly set but still a bit wet on top, sprinkle the Parmesan cheese (if using) over half of the omelette.

7. Fold the plain half of the omelette over the cheese half. Slide the omelette onto a plate and serve immediately.

This mushroom and spinach omelette is an excellent choice for young men aiming for weight loss for a few reasons:

- Eggs are a lean, high•protein food that helps keep you feeling full.
- Mushrooms and spinach add fiber, vitamins, and minerals without a lot of calories.
- The portion size is reasonable and satisfying, without going overboard on calories.

Pair this omelette with a side of fresh fruit or a small whole grain toast for a complete, nutrient•dense meal. Enjoy!

62. Greek Yogurt Smoothie

Ingredient:

• 1 cup plain Greek yogurt
• 1 cup unsweetened almond milk (or milk of your choice)
• 1 cup frozen mixed berries (such as blueberries, raspberries, strawberries)
• 1 tbsp honey (optional)
• 1 tsp vanilla extract
• 1/4 tsp ground cinnamon (optional)
• Ice cubes (optional)

Instructions:

1. In a high•powered blender, combine the Greek yogurt, almond milk, frozen berries, honey (if using), vanilla extract, and cinnamon (if using).

2. Blend on high speed until the mixture is smooth and creamy, about 1•2 minutes.

3. If you'd like a thicker, colder smoothie, add a few ice cubes and blend again briefly.

4. Pour the Greek yogurt smoothie into a glass and enjoy immediately.

This smoothie is an excellent choice for a healthy snack or light meal. Here's why it's great for health and weight loss:

• Greek yogurt is high in protein, which helps keep you feeling full and satisfied.
• Berries are packed with fiber, vitamins, and antioxidants.
• Almond milk is low in calories and provides a creamy texture without the fat of regular milk.
• Honey and cinnamon are optional additions that can provide natural sweetness and health benefits.

You can customize this smoothie by using different types of fruit, adding a handful of spinach or kale, or using a plant•based protein powder. It's a versatile and nutritious way to start your day or refuel after a workout.

Enjoy your Greek yogurt smoothie!

63. Chicken and Chickpea Salad

Ingredient:

• 2 cups cooked and shredded chicken breast
• 1 (15 oz) can chickpeas, drained and rinsed
• 1 cup diced cucumber
• 1/2 cup diced red onion
• 1/2 cup halved cherry tomatoes
• 2 tbsp chopped fresh parsley
• 2 tbsp lemon juice
• 1 tbsp olive oil
• 1 tsp Dijon mustard
• 1/4 tsp salt
• 1/4 tsp black pepper

Instructions:

1. In a large bowl, combine the shredded chicken, chickpeas, diced cucumber, red onion, cherry tomatoes, and chopped parsley.

2. In a small bowl, whisk together the lemon juice, olive oil, Dijon mustard, salt, and black pepper to make the dressing.

3. Pour the dressing over the chicken and chickpea mixture and toss gently to coat everything evenly.

4. Serve the chicken and chickpea salad chilled or at room temperature. It can be enjoyed on its own or over a bed of mixed greens.

This salad is an excellent choice for young men aiming for weight loss for a few reasons:

• Chicken is a lean protein that helps keep you feeling full and satisfied.
• Chickpeas are a good source of fiber, protein, and complex carbohydrates.
• The fresh vegetables add volume, fiber, and antioxidants without a lot of calories.
• The simple dressing is light and flavorful without weighing down the dish.

This salad makes for a satisfying and nutritious meal or snack that can support weight loss goals. It's easy to prepare and can be made ahead of time for quick lunches or dinners. Enjoy!

64. Spicy Lentil Patties

Ingredient:

• 1 cup cooked brown or green lentils
• 1/2 cup rolled oats
• 1/4 cup finely chopped onion
• 2 cloves garlic, minced
• 1 tsp ground cumin
• 1 tsp chili powder
• 1/4 tsp cayenne pepper (or to taste)
• 1/4 tsp salt
• 1 tbsp olive oil

Instructions:

1. In a medium bowl, mash the cooked lentils with a fork or potato masher until slightly chunky.

2. Add the rolled oats, chopped onion, minced garlic, cumin, chili powder, cayenne pepper, and salt. Mix well until fully combined.

3. Divide the lentil mixture into 6 equal portions and shape each one into a patty, about 1/2 inch thick.

4. Heat the olive oil in a large non•stick skillet over medium heat.

5. Working in batches if needed, add the lentil patties to the hot skillet and cook for 3•4 minutes per side, until golden brown and crispy.

6. Carefully transfer the cooked lentil patties to a plate or baking sheet.

7. Serve the spicy lentil patties warm, either on their own or on a bun with your favorite toppings like avocado, tomato, or lettuce.

These lentil patties are a great meatless option that are high in protein, fiber, and complex carbohydrates. The spices add a nice kick of flavor. They can be enjoyed as a main dish, a burger alternative, or even as a snack.

Lentils are an excellent choice for young men aiming for weight loss, as they are filling and nutrient•dense without a lot of calories. Pair these patties with a fresh salad or roasted vegetables for a complete, balanced meal.

65. Broccoli and Almond Stir•Fry

Ingredient:

- 1 lb broccoli florets, cut into bite•sized pieces
- 2 tbsp olive oil
- 3 cloves garlic, minced
- 1 inch piece fresh ginger, peeled and grated
- 1/4 cup sliced almonds
- 2 tbsp low•sodium soy sauce or tamari
- 1 tsp sesame oil
- 1/4 tsp red pepper flakes (optional)
- Salt and black pepper to taste
- Chopped green onions for garnish (optional)

Instructions:

1. Heat the olive oil in a large skillet or wok over medium•high heat.

2. Add the broccoli florets and stir•fry for 3•4 minutes, until they start to soften and char slightly.

3. Add the minced garlic and grated ginger. Stir•fry for 1 minute until fragrant.

4. Stir in the sliced almonds and continue stir•frying for 2•3 minutes, until the almonds are lightly toasted.

5. Pour in the soy sauce and sesame oil. Toss everything together and cook for 1•2 minutes more.

6. Remove from heat and season with salt, black pepper, and red pepper flakes (if using).

7. Transfer the broccoli and almond stir•fry to a serving dish. Garnish with chopped green onions if desired.

Serve this stir•fry hot, either on its own or over a bed of steamed brown rice or quinoa. The broccoli provides fiber, vitamins, and minerals, while the almonds add a satisfying crunch and healthy fats. This dish is low in calories but high in nutrients, making it an excellent choice for a healthy meal.

Enjoy!

66. Roasted Red Pepper Hummus

Ingredient:

• 1 (15 oz) can chickpeas, drained and rinsed
• 1/2 cup roasted red peppers, drained and patted dry
• 2 tbsp tahini
• 2 tbsp fresh lemon juice
• 2 cloves garlic, minced
• 1 tsp ground cumin
• 1/4 tsp cayenne pepper (optional)
• 2•3 tbsp water, as needed
• Salt and black pepper to taste
• Chopped parsley for garnish (optional)

Instructions:

1. In a food processor or high•powered blender, combine the drained and rinsed chickpeas, roasted red peppers, tahini, lemon juice, minced garlic, cumin, and cayenne pepper (if using).

2. Pulse the mixture several times, then process or blend on high speed, scraping down the sides as needed, until the hummus is smooth and creamy.

3. If the hummus seems too thick, add 1•2 tablespoons of water and blend again until you reach your desired consistency.

4. Season the roasted red pepper hummus with salt and black pepper to taste.

5. Transfer the hummus to a serving bowl and garnish with chopped parsley, if desired.

6. Serve the hummus with fresh vegetables, whole grain crackers, or pita bread for dipping.

This roasted red pepper hummus is a nutritious and flavorful snack or appetizer that's perfect for young men aiming for weight loss. Chickpeas are high in protein and fiber, while the roasted red peppers add a sweet and smoky element. The tahini provides healthy fats to help keep you feeling full.

You can adjust the amount of cayenne pepper to control the level of spiciness. This hummus can also be customized by adding other roasted vegetables, fresh herbs, or spices to suit your taste preferences.

67. Tuna and Quinoa Salad

Ingredient:

- 1 cup cooked quinoa, cooled
- 1 (5 oz) can tuna, drained and flaked
- 1 cup diced cucumber
- 1/2 cup diced cherry tomatoes
- 1/4 cup diced red onion
- 2 tbsp chopped fresh parsley
- 2 tbsp lemon juice
- 1 tbsp olive oil
- 1/4 tsp salt
- 1/4 tsp black pepper

Instructions:

1. In a large bowl, combine the cooked quinoa, flaked tuna, diced cucumber, cherry tomatoes, red onion, and chopped parsley.

2. In a small bowl, whisk together the lemon juice, olive oil, salt, and pepper.

3. Pour the dressing over the quinoa and tuna mixture and toss gently to coat everything evenly.

4. Serve the tuna and quinoa salad chilled or at room temperature. It can be enjoyed on its own or over a bed of mixed greens.

This salad is an excellent choice for young men aiming for weight loss for a few reasons:

- Quinoa is a high•protein, high•fiber grain that helps keep you feeling full.
- Tuna is a lean protein that is low in calories and fat, but high in nutrients like omega•3s.
- The fresh vegetables add volume, fiber, and antioxidants without a lot of calories.
- The simple dressing is light and flavorful without weighing down the dish.

This salad makes for a satisfying and nutritious meal or snack that can support weight loss goals. It's easy to prepare and can be made ahead of time for quick lunches or dinners. Enjoy!

68. Eggplant and Tomato Bake

Ingredient:

- 1 medium eggplant, sliced into 1/2•inch rounds
- 2 tbsp olive oil, divided
- 1 onion, diced
- 3 cloves garlic, minced
- 1 (14.5 oz) can diced tomatoes
- 1 tsp dried oregano
- 1/2 tsp dried basil
- 1/4 tsp red pepper flakes (optional)
- Salt and black pepper to taste
- 1 cup shredded mozzarella cheese

Instructions:

1. Preheat your oven to 375°F (190°C). Lightly grease a 9x13 inch baking dish.

2. Arrange the eggplant slices in a single layer on a baking sheet. Brush both sides with 1 tbsp of the olive oil. Bake for 15•20 minutes, flipping halfway, until the eggplant is tender.

3. In a skillet, heat the remaining 1 tbsp of olive oil over medium heat. Add the diced onion and sauté for 3•4 minutes until translucent.

4. Add the minced garlic and cook for 1 minute more, until fragrant.

5. Stir in the diced tomatoes, dried oregano, dried basil, and red pepper flakes (if using). Season with salt and black pepper to taste.

6. Arrange the baked eggplant slices in the prepared baking dish. Pour the tomato mixture over the top and spread it evenly.

7. Sprinkle the shredded mozzarella cheese over the top.

8. Bake the eggplant and tomato bake for 20•25 minutes, until the cheese is melted and bubbly. Let the dish cool for 5 minutes before serving.

This eggplant and tomato bake is a delicious and healthy vegetarian dish that's perfect for young men aiming for weight loss. The eggplant and tomatoes provide fiber, vitamins, and antioxidants, while the cheese adds a satisfying creaminess. Enjoy!

69. Spicy Grilled Chicken Thighs

Ingredient:

- 8 boneless, skinless chicken thighs
- 2 tbsp olive oil
- 2 tsp chili powder
- 1 tsp smoked paprika
- 1 tsp garlic powder
- 1/2 tsp onion powder
- 1/2 tsp cayenne pepper (or to taste)
- 1 tsp salt
- 1/2 tsp black pepper

Instructions:

1. In a large bowl, combine the chicken thighs, olive oil, chili powder, smoked paprika, garlic powder, onion powder, cayenne pepper, salt, and black pepper. Toss to coat the chicken evenly.

2. Preheat your grill or grill pan to medium·high heat.

3. Grill the chicken thighs for 5·7 minutes per side, or until they reach an internal temperature of 165°F (75°C).

4. Transfer the grilled chicken thighs to a clean plate and let them rest for 5 minutes before serving.

These spicy grilled chicken thighs are a great option for young men aiming for weight loss for a few reasons:

- Chicken thighs are a lean protein that is more affordable and flavorful than chicken breasts.
- The spices add bold flavor without the need for high·calorie sauces or marinades.
- Grilling the chicken is a healthy cooking method that doesn't require added fats.
- Chicken thighs are more satisfying and filling than chicken breasts, which can help with hunger management.

Serve the spicy grilled chicken thighs with a side of roasted vegetables or a fresh salad for a complete, nutrient·dense meal. The bold flavors and tender texture of the chicken will make this a family·friendly dish that supports your weight loss goals.

70. Zoodles with Tomato Sauce

Ingredient:

• 3 medium zucchinis, spiralized or julienned into noodles
• 1 tbsp olive oil
• 1 garlic clove, minced
• 1 (14.5 oz) can diced tomatoes
• 2 tbsp tomato paste
• 1 tsp dried oregano
• 1/4 tsp red pepper flakes (optional)
• Salt and black pepper to taste
• Grated Parmesan cheese for serving (optional)
• Chopped fresh basil for garnish (optional)

Instructions:

1. Using a spiralizer, julienne slicer, or vegetable peeler, cut the zucchinis into long, thin noodle•like strips (zoodles).

2. In a large skillet, heat the olive oil over medium heat. Add the minced garlic and sauté for 1 minute until fragrant.

3. Add the diced tomatoes, tomato paste, dried oregano, and red pepper flakes (if using). Season with salt and black pepper to taste.

4. Bring the tomato sauce to a simmer and let it cook for 5•7 minutes, stirring occasionally, until slightly thickened.

5. Add the zucchini noodles to the skillet and toss to coat them evenly with the tomato sauce. Cook for 2•3 minutes, just until the zoodles are tender but still have a bit of bite.

6. Remove the zoodles and tomato sauce from heat. Serve the zoodles warm, topped with grated Parmesan cheese and chopped fresh basil, if desired.

This zoodles with tomato sauce dish is a delicious and healthy alternative to traditional pasta. Zucchini noodles are low in calories and carbs, making them a great option for young men alming for weight loss. The simple tomato sauce provides flavor and nutrients without the heaviness of a cream•based sauce.

You can customize this recipe by adding other vegetables, lean proteins, or herbs to suit your taste preferences. Enjoy this light and satisfying zoodle dish!

71. Cabbage and Carrot Slaw

Ingredient:

- 1/2 head green cabbage, shredded (about 4 cups)
- 2 carrots, peeled and grated (about 1 cup)
- 1/2 red onion, thinly sliced
- 2 tbsp apple cider vinegar
- 1 tbsp Dijon mustard
- 1 tbsp honey
- 2 tbsp olive oil
- Salt and black pepper to taste
- 2 tbsp chopped fresh parsley (optional)

Instructions:

1. In a large bowl, combine the shredded cabbage, grated carrots, and sliced red onion.

2. In a small bowl, whisk together the apple cider vinegar, Dijon mustard, honey, and olive oil. Season with salt and pepper.

3. Pour the dressing over the cabbage and carrot mixture and toss to coat everything evenly.

4. Let the slaw sit for 10•15 minutes to allow the flavors to meld.

5. Just before serving, stir in the chopped fresh parsley, if using.

This cabbage and carrot slaw makes a great side dish or topping for sandwiches, tacos, or burgers. It's packed with fiber, vitamins, and antioxidants from the vegetables. The tangy•sweet dressing complements the crunchy texture perfectly.

Some variations you could try:
- Add thinly sliced radishes or jicama for extra crunch
- Sprinkle in some toasted sunflower or pumpkin seeds
- Use a mix of green and red cabbage for more color
- Swap the honey for maple syrup or agave nectar

Enjoy this healthy and flavorful slaw!

72. Salmon and Avocado Salad

Ingredient:

- 1 (6 oz) salmon fillet, cooked and flaked
- 1 avocado, diced
- 1 cup cherry tomatoes, halved
- 1/2 cup diced cucumber
- 2 tbsp chopped red onion
- 2 tbsp chopped fresh cilantro
- 1 tbsp olive oil
- 1 tbsp lemon juice
- 1/4 tsp salt
- 1/4 tsp black pepper

Instructions:

1. In a large bowl, gently combine the flaked cooked salmon, diced avocado, cherry tomatoes, diced cucumber, red onion, and chopped cilantro.

2. In a small bowl, whisk together the olive oil, lemon juice, salt, and black pepper to make the dressing.

3. Pour the dressing over the salmon and avocado mixture and toss gently to coat.

4. Serve the salmon and avocado salad chilled or at room temperature. It can be enjoyed on its own or over a bed of mixed greens.

This salad is an excellent choice for young men aiming for weight loss for a few reasons:

- Salmon is a lean protein that is high in omega•3 fatty acids, which are beneficial for heart health.
- Avocado provides healthy fats and fiber to help keep you feeling full.
- The fresh vegetables add volume, fiber, and antioxidants without a lot of calories.
- The simple dressing is light and flavorful without weighing down the dish.

This salad makes for a satisfying and nutritious meal or snack that can support weight loss goals. The combination of salmon, avocado, and fresh produce creates a well•balanced and delicious dish.

73. Roasted Beet and Goat Cheese Salad

Ingredient:

- 3 medium beets, peeled and cut into 1·inch cubes
- 2 tbsp olive oil
- Salt and black pepper to taste
- 5 oz mixed greens
- 2 oz crumbled goat cheese
- 2 tbsp toasted walnuts or pecans
- 2 tbsp balsamic vinegar
- 1 tbsp honey

Instructions:

1. Preheat your oven to 400°F (200°C). Line a baking sheet with parchment paper.

2. In a bowl, toss the cubed beets with the olive oil and season with salt and pepper.

3. Spread the seasoned beets in a single layer on the prepared baking sheet.

4. Roast the beets for 25·30 minutes, stirring halfway, until they are tender and lightly caramelized.

5. Remove the roasted beets from the oven and let them cool slightly.

6. In a large salad bowl, combine the mixed greens, roasted beets, crumbled goat cheese, and toasted nuts.

7. In a small bowl, whisk together the balsamic vinegar and honey to make the dressing. Drizzle the balsamic dressing over the salad and toss gently to coat. Serve the roasted beet and goat cheese salad immediately.

This salad is a great option for young men aiming for weight loss for a few reasons:

- Beets are low in calories but high in fiber, vitamins, and antioxidants.
- Goat cheese provides a creamy, tangy element with a moderate amount of healthy fats.
- The mixed greens and toasted nuts add crunch and additional nutrients.
- The balsamic·honey dressing is light and flavorful without being heavy.

This salad makes for a satisfying and nutritious meal or side dish. The combination of flavors and textures is both delicious and visually appealing. Enjoy this roasted beet and goat cheese salad!

74. Turkey and Spinach Meatloaf

Ingredient:

• 1 lb ground turkey
• 1 cup chopped fresh spinach
• 1/2 cup diced onion
• 2 cloves garlic, minced
• 1/2 cup whole wheat breadcrumbs
• 1 egg
• 2 tbsp tomato paste
• 1 tsp dried oregano
• 1/2 tsp salt
• 1/4 tsp black pepper

Instructions:

1. Preheat your oven to 375°F (190°C). Lightly grease a 9x5 inch loaf pan.

2. In a large bowl, combine the ground turkey, chopped spinach, diced onion, minced garlic, whole wheat breadcrumbs, egg, tomato paste, oregano, salt, and black pepper. Mix until all the ingredients are well incorporated.

3. Transfer the turkey and spinach mixture to the prepared loaf pan, gently pressing it down to compact it.

4. Bake the meatloaf for 45·55 minutes, until the internal temperature reaches 165°F (75°C).

5. Remove the meatloaf from the oven and let it rest for 5·10 minutes before slicing and serving.

This turkey and spinach meatloaf is an excellent choice for young men aiming for weight loss for a few reasons:

• Ground turkey is a lean protein that is lower in fat and calories compared to ground beef.
• Spinach adds fiber, vitamins, and minerals without a lot of calories.
• Whole wheat breadcrumbs provide complex carbohydrates to help keep you feeling full.
• The simple seasoning allows the natural flavors of the ingredients to shine through.

Serve this meatloaf with roasted vegetables or a fresh salad for a complete, nutrient·dense meal. The leftovers also make a great option for quick lunches or dinners throughout the week

75. Steamed Mussels with Garlic

Ingredient:

• 2 lbs mussels, scrubbed and debearded
• 2 tbsp olive oil
• 4 cloves garlic, minced
• 1/2 cup dry white wine or low•sodium chicken/vegetable broth
• 1 tbsp lemon juice
• 2 tbsp chopped fresh parsley
• Salt and black pepper to taste
• Lemon wedges for serving

Instructions:

1. In a large pot or Dutch oven, heat the olive oil over medium heat. Add the minced garlic and sauté for 1 minute until fragrant.

2. Add the mussels to the pot and pour in the white wine or broth. Cover the pot with a lid and steam the mussels for 5•7 minutes, until they have all opened up.

3. Discard any mussels that did not open.

4. Stir in the lemon juice and chopped parsley. Season with salt and black pepper to taste.

5. Serve the steamed mussels immediately, with lemon wedges on the side.

This steamed mussels dish is an excellent choice for young men aiming for weight loss for a few reasons:

• Mussels are a lean, low•calorie protein source that is high in nutrients like vitamin B12, iron, and omega•3 fatty acids.
• The simple garlic and white wine/broth preparation allows the natural flavors of the mussels to shine through without adding a lot of extra calories.
• Lemon juice provides a bright, tangy contrast that enhances the dish without the need for heavy sauces.
• Mussels are very filling, so this can make for a satisfying meal without going overboard on calories.

Serve the steamed mussels with a side of roasted vegetables or a fresh salad for a complete, nutrient•dense meal. Enjoy this delicious and healthy seafood dish!

76. Grilled Asparagus with Lemon

Ingredient:

• 1 lb asparagus, woody ends trimmed
• 2 tbsp olive oil
• 1 tbsp lemon juice
• 1 tsp grated lemon zest
• 1/4 tsp salt
• 1/4 tsp black pepper

Instructions:

1. Preheat your grill or grill pan to medium•high heat.

2. In a large bowl, toss the trimmed asparagus spears with the olive oil, lemon juice, lemon zest, salt, and black pepper until the asparagus is evenly coated.

3. Arrange the seasoned asparagus in a single layer on the hot grill or grill pan.

4. Grill the asparagus for 5•7 minutes, turning occasionally, until it's tender and lightly charred.

5. Transfer the grilled asparagus to a serving platter or plate.

6. Serve the grilled asparagus with lemon wedges on the side, allowing people to squeeze additional lemon juice over the top if desired.

This grilled asparagus with lemon is a simple yet flavorful side dish that's perfect for young men aiming for weight loss. Here's why it's a great option:

• Asparagus is low in calories but high in fiber, vitamins, and antioxidants.
• Grilling the asparagus adds a delicious smoky flavor without the need for heavy sauces or toppings.
• The lemon juice and zest provide a bright, refreshing contrast to the grilled asparagus.
• This dish is easy to prepare and pairs well with a variety of main courses, from grilled chicken to roasted salmon.

You can customize this recipe by adding a sprinkle of Parmesan cheese, toasted nuts, or fresh herbs. Enjoy this healthy and tasty grilled asparagus with lemon!

77. Chicken and Mushroom Stir•Fry

Ingredient:

- 1 lb boneless, skinless chicken breasts, cut into 1•inch pieces
- 2 tbsp low•sodium soy sauce
- 1 tbsp rice vinegar
- 1 tsp sesame oil
- 1 tbsp cornstarch
- 2 tbsp olive oil
- 8 oz sliced mushrooms
- 1 red bell pepper, sliced
- 3 cloves garlic, minced
- 1 tbsp grated fresh ginger
- 2 cups cooked brown rice, for serving

Instructions:

1. In a medium bowl, combine the chicken, soy sauce, rice vinegar, sesame oil, and cornstarch. Toss to coat the chicken and let it marinate for 15•20 minutes.

2. Heat the olive oil in a large skillet or wok over high heat.

3. Add the marinated chicken and stir•fry for 3•4 minutes, until the chicken is lightly browned.

4. Add the sliced mushrooms and red bell pepper. Stir•fry for 3•4 minutes, until the vegetables are tender•crisp.

5. Stir in the minced garlic and grated ginger. Cook for 1 minute, until fragrant.

6. Serve the chicken and mushroom stir•fry immediately over the cooked brown rice.

This chicken and mushroom stir•fry is a great option for young men aiming for weight loss for a few reasons:

- Chicken breast is a lean protein that is low in fat and calories.
- Mushrooms and bell peppers add fiber, vitamins, and minerals without a lot of calories.
- The stir•fry cooking method uses minimal oil, keeping the dish light and healthy.
- Serving the stir•fry over brown rice provides complex carbohydrates to help keep you feeling full.

78. Stuffed Zucchini Boats

Ingredient:

• 4 medium zucchinis, halved lengthwise
• 1 tbsp olive oil
• 1 lb ground turkey or lean ground beef
• 1 onion, diced
• 2 cloves garlic, minced
• 1 tsp dried oregano
• 1/2 tsp dried basil
• 1/4 tsp red pepper flakes (optional)
• 1 (14.5 oz) can diced tomatoes
• 1/2 cup shredded mozzarella cheese
• Salt and black pepper to taste
• Chopped fresh parsley for garnish (optional)

Instructions:

1. Preheat your oven to 375°F (190°C). Scoop out the flesh from the zucchini halves, leaving about 1/4 inch of the zucchini shell. Finely chop the scooped•out zucchini flesh.

2. In a large skillet, heat the olive oil over medium heat. Add the ground turkey/beef and cook, breaking it up with a spatula, until browned, about 5•7 minutes.

3. Add the diced onion, minced garlic, chopped zucchini flesh, oregano, basil, and red pepper flakes (if using). Cook for 3•4 minutes, stirring occasionally, until the vegetables are softened.

4. Stir in the diced tomatoes and season with salt and black pepper to taste. Simmer the mixture for 5•7 minutes, allowing the flavors to meld.

5. Arrange the zucchini boat halves in a baking dish. Spoon the turkey/beef mixture evenly into the zucchini boats.

6. Top the stuffed zucchini boats with the shredded mozzarella cheese.

7. Bake the stuffed zucchini for 20•25 minutes, until the zucchini is tender and the cheese is melted and bubbly. Garnish the stuffed zucchini boats with chopped fresh parsley, if desired.

These stuffed zucchini boats are a delicious and healthy meal option. The lean ground turkey or beef provides protein, while the zucchini and tomatoes add fiber and nutrients. This dish is a great way to incorporate more vegetables into your diet.

79. Cucumber and Mint Salad

Ingredient:

- 2 medium cucumbers, sliced
- 1/2 red onion, thinly sliced
- 1/4 cup chopped fresh mint leaves
- 2 tbsp olive oil
- 1 tbsp white wine vinegar
- 1 tbsp lemon juice
- 1/4 tsp salt
- 1/4 tsp black pepper

Instructions:

1. In a large bowl, combine the sliced cucumbers, thinly sliced red onion, and chopped fresh mint leaves.

2. In a small bowl, whisk together the olive oil, white wine vinegar, lemon juice, salt, and black pepper to make the dressing.

3. Pour the dressing over the cucumber and mint mixture and toss gently to coat everything evenly.

4. Cover the salad and refrigerate for at least 30 minutes to allow the flavors to meld.

5. Serve the chilled cucumber and mint salad as a refreshing side dish.

This cucumber and mint salad is a great option for young men aiming for weight loss for a few reasons:

- Cucumbers are low in calories but high in water content, which can help you feel full.
- The fresh mint adds a bright, aromatic flavor without the need for heavy dressings or sauces.
- The simple olive oil and vinegar dressing is light and flavorful without weighing down the dish.
- This salad is easy to prepare and can be made ahead of time for quick, healthy meals.

You can customize this recipe by adding other fresh herbs, such as dill or parsley, or by including halved cherry tomatoes or crumbled feta cheese.

Enjoy this refreshing and nutritious Cucumber and Mint Salad!

80. Grilled Pineapple with Chicken

Ingredient:

• 1 lb boneless, skinless chicken breasts
• 1 fresh pineapple, cut into 1•inch thick slices
• 2 tbsp olive oil
• 1 tbsp honey
• 1 tsp chili powder
• 1/2 tsp garlic powder
• 1/4 tsp salt
• 1/4 tsp black pepper

Instructions:

1. Preheat your grill or grill pan to medium•high heat.

2. In a small bowl, whisk together the olive oil, honey, chili powder, garlic powder, salt, and black pepper to make the marinade.

3. Place the chicken breasts and pineapple slices in a large resealable bag or shallow dish. Pour the marinade over the top and toss to coat everything evenly.

4. Grill the chicken and pineapple for 5•7 minutes per side, or until the chicken is cooked through and the pineapple is lightly charred.

5. Remove the grilled chicken and pineapple from the heat and let them rest for a few minutes.

6. Slice the grilled chicken breasts and serve them alongside the grilled pineapple slices.

This grilled pineapple with chicken dish is an excellent choice for young men aiming for weight loss for a few reasons:

• Chicken breast is a lean protein that is low in fat and calories.
• Pineapple is a sweet, juicy fruit that is high in fiber and vitamins, but low in calories.
• The marinade adds flavor without the need for high•calorie sauces or dressings.
• Grilling the chicken and pineapple is a healthy cooking method that doesn't require added fats.

Serve this dish with a side of roasted vegetables or a fresh salad for a complete, nutrient•dense meal. The sweet and savory flavors of the grilled pineapple and chicken make this a delicious and satisfying option for weight loss.

81. Roasted Garlic Cauliflower

Ingredient:

• 1 head of cauliflower, cut into florets
• 3 tbsp olive oil
• 4 cloves garlic, minced
• 1 tsp dried thyme
• 1/2 tsp salt
• 1/4 tsp black pepper
• 2 tbsp grated Parmesan cheese (optional)
• Chopped parsley for garnish (optional)

Instructions:

1. Preheat your oven to 400°F (200°C). Line a large baking sheet with parchment paper.

2. In a large bowl, toss the cauliflower florets with the olive oil, minced garlic, dried thyme, salt, and black pepper until the cauliflower is evenly coated.

3. Spread the seasoned cauliflower in a single layer on the prepared baking sheet.

4. Roast the cauliflower for 20•25 minutes, stirring halfway, until it's tender and lightly browned.

5. Remove the roasted cauliflower from the oven and sprinkle with the grated Parmesan cheese, if using.

6. Serve the roasted garlic cauliflower warm, garnished with chopped parsley if desired.

This roasted garlic cauliflower makes a delicious and healthy side dish or snack. The combination of roasted garlic, thyme, and Parmesan (if using) adds tons of flavor to the cauliflower.

Cauliflower is an excellent choice for young men aiming for weight loss. It's low in calories but high in fiber, vitamins, and minerals. The roasting process also brings out the natural sweetness of the cauliflower.

You can customize this recipe by adding other spices, herbs, or a squeeze of lemon juice. Serve the roasted garlic cauliflower alongside grilled chicken, fish, or as part of a vegetarian meal.

82. Spicy Chickpea and Spinach Stew

Ingredient:

- 2 tbsp olive oil
- 1 onion, diced
- 3 cloves garlic, minced
- 1 tbsp grated ginger
- 1 tsp ground cumin
- 1 tsp smoked paprika
- 1/2 tsp cayenne pepper (or to taste)
- 1 (15oz) can diced tomatoes
- 1 (15oz) can chickpeas, drained and rinsed
- 4 cups vegetable or chicken broth
- 5 oz baby spinach
- Salt and pepper to taste
- Chopped cilantro for serving

Instructions:

1. In a large pot or Dutch oven, heat the olive oil over medium heat. Add the onion and sauté for 5 minutes until translucent.

2. Add the garlic, ginger, cumin, paprika, and cayenne. Cook for 1 minute, stirring constantly, until fragrant.

3. Pour in the diced tomatoes with their juices and the chickpeas. Stir to combine.

4. Add the broth and bring the stew to a simmer. Reduce heat and let simmer for 15•20 minutes.

5. Stir in the baby spinach and cook for 2•3 minutes until the spinach is wilted.

6. Season with salt and pepper to taste.

7. Serve the spicy chickpea and spinach stew hot, garnished with chopped cilantro.

This hearty, vegetarian stew is packed with protein from the chickpeas and nutrients from the spinach. The spices give it a nice kick of flavor.

83. Salmon and Sweet Potato Cakes

Ingredient:

- 1 lb salmon fillets, cooked and flaked
- 1 medium sweet potato, peeled and grated (about 1 cup grated)
- 1/4 cup all•purpose flour
- 1 egg, beaten
- 2 tbsp chopped fresh parsley
- 1 tsp lemon zest
- 1/2 tsp salt
- 1/4 tsp black pepper
- 2 tbsp olive oil

Instructions:

1. In a large bowl, combine the flaked salmon, grated sweet potato, flour, egg, parsley, lemon zest, salt, and pepper. Mix well until fully incorporated.

2. Form the mixture into 8 equal•sized patties, about 1/2 inch thick.

3. Heat the olive oil in a large skillet over medium heat.

4. Working in batches if needed, cook the salmon and sweet potato cakes for 3•4 minutes per side, until golden brown.

5. Drain the cakes on a paper towel•lined plate.

6. Serve the salmon and sweet potato cakes warm, with desired toppings or sauces.

Enjoy these delicious and healthy salmon and sweet potato cakes! The sweet potato adds a nice texture and flavor to the salmon patties.

84. Avocado and Black Bean Salad

Ingredient:

• 1 (15 oz) can black beans, drained and rinsed
• 1 avocado, diced
• 1 cup cherry tomatoes, halved
• 1/2 cup diced red onion
• 1/4 cup chopped fresh cilantro
• 2 tbsp lime juice
• 1 tbsp olive oil
• 1/4 tsp ground cumin
• 1/4 tsp salt
• 1/4 tsp black pepper

Instructions:

1. In a large bowl, combine the drained and rinsed black beans, diced avocado, halved cherry tomatoes, diced red onion, and chopped fresh cilantro.

2. In a small bowl, whisk together the lime juice, olive oil, ground cumin, salt, and black pepper to make the dressing.

3. Pour the dressing over the black bean and avocado mixture and toss gently to coat everything evenly.

4. Serve the avocado and black bean salad chilled or at room temperature.

This salad is an excellent choice for young men aiming for weight loss for a few reasons:

• Black beans are a great source of plant•based protein and fiber, which can help keep you feeling full.
• Avocado provides healthy fats and creaminess to the salad without a lot of calories.
• The fresh vegetables add volume, fiber, and antioxidants without a lot of calories.
• The simple lime•based dressing is light and flavorful without weighing down the dish.

This salad makes for a satisfying and nutritious meal or snack that can support weight loss goals. It's easy to prepare and can be made ahead of time for quick lunches or dinners. Enjoy this delicious and healthy Avocado and Black Bean Salad!

85. Sautéed Spinach with Garlic

Ingredient:

- 1 lb fresh spinach, washed and stems removed
- 2 tbsp olive oil
- 3 cloves garlic, minced
- 1/4 tsp red pepper flakes (optional)
- 1/4 tsp salt
- 1/8 tsp black pepper

Instructions:

1. In a large skillet or wok, heat the olive oil over medium heat.

2. Add the minced garlic and sauté for 1 minute, until fragrant.

3. Add the fresh spinach to the skillet in batches, stirring constantly, until the spinach is wilted down, about 2•3 minutes per batch.

4. Once all the spinach has been added and wilted, sprinkle in the red pepper flakes (if using), salt, and black pepper. Toss to combine.

5. Continue to sauté the spinach for 1•2 minutes more, until heated through.

6. Serve the sautéed spinach with garlic warm, as a side dish.

This sautéed spinach with garlic is a simple yet flavorful way to enjoy this nutrient•dense green. It's an excellent option for young men aiming for weight loss for a few reasons:

- Spinach is low in calories but high in fiber, vitamins, and minerals.
- Garlic adds bold flavor without the need for heavy sauces or seasonings.
- The sautéing method cooks the spinach quickly, preserving its nutrients.
- This dish is easy to prepare and can be enjoyed as a side or incorporated into other meals.

You can customize this recipe by adding a squeeze of lemon juice, a sprinkle of Parmesan cheese, or a drizzle of balsamic glaze. Sautéed spinach with garlic pairs well with grilled chicken, roasted salmon, or as a topping for whole grain dishes.

Enjoy this simple and nutritious sautéed spinach side dish!

86. Baked Herb•Crusted Tilapia

Ingredient:

• 4 tilapia fillets (about 1 lb total)
• 1/2 cup panko breadcrumbs
• 2 tbsp grated Parmesan cheese
• 1 tsp dried parsley
• 1 tsp dried basil
• 1/2 tsp garlic powder
• 1/4 tsp salt
• 1/4 tsp black pepper
• 1 tbsp olive oil

Instructions:

1. Preheat oven to 400°F. Line a baking sheet with parchment paper.

2. In a shallow bowl, mix together the panko, Parmesan, parsley, basil, garlic powder, salt, and pepper.

3. Brush the tilapia fillets lightly with the olive oil on both sides.

4. Dip the tilapia into the breadcrumb mixture, pressing gently to help it adhere.

5. Place the coated tilapia fillets on the prepared baking sheet.

6. Bake for 12•15 minutes, until the fish flakes easily with a fork and the breadcrumbs are golden brown.

This recipe is a great option for weight loss as tilapia is a lean, low•calorie protein source. The herb•crusted topping adds flavor without a lot of extra calories or fat. Serve with a side of roasted vegetables for a complete, healthy meal.

87. Lentil and Carrot Soup

Ingredient:

- 1 tbsp olive oil
- 1 onion, diced
- 3 carrots, peeled and diced
- 3 cloves garlic, minced
- 1 tsp ground cumin
- 1 tsp dried thyme
- 1/4 tsp cayenne pepper (optional)
- 1 cup brown or green lentils, rinsed
- 4 cups low•sodium vegetable or chicken broth
- 1 (14.5 oz) can diced tomatoes
- 2 cups baby spinach or kale, chopped
- Salt and black pepper to taste

Instructions:

1. In a large pot or Dutch oven, heat the olive oil over medium heat. Add the onion and carrots and cook for 5•7 minutes until softened.

2. Add the garlic, cumin, thyme, and cayenne (if using). Cook for 1 minute until fragrant.

3. Stir in the lentils, broth, and diced tomatoes. Bring to a boil, then reduce heat and simmer for 20•25 minutes, until the lentils are tender.

4. Stir in the spinach or kale and cook for 2•3 minutes until wilted.

5. Season with salt and pepper to taste.

This lentil and carrot soup is packed with fiber, protein, and nutrients to keep you feeling full and satisfied. The lentils provide a hearty, filling base, while the carrots and greens add vitamins and antioxidants. It's a simple, wholesome soup that's perfect for weight loss.

88. Chicken and Green Bean Stir•Fry

Ingredient:

• 1 lb boneless, skinless chicken breasts, cut into 1•inch pieces
• 1 tbsp sesame oil
• 2 cloves garlic, minced
• 1 tbsp grated fresh ginger
• 1 lb green beans, trimmed and cut into 1•inch pieces
• 2 tbsp low•sodium soy sauce
• 1 tbsp rice vinegar
• 1 tsp honey
• 1/4 tsp red pepper flakes (optional)
• Salt and black pepper to taste
• 2 cups cooked brown rice, for serving

Instructions:

1. Heat the sesame oil in a large skillet or wok over high heat. Add the chicken and cook for 3•4 minutes, until lightly browned.

2. Add the garlic and ginger and cook for 1 minute, until fragrant.

3. Add the green beans and stir•fry for 4•5 minutes, until the beans are tender•crisp.

4. In a small bowl, whisk together the soy sauce, rice vinegar, honey, and red pepper flakes (if using).

5. Pour the sauce into the skillet and toss everything together until the chicken is cooked through and the sauce has thickened slightly, about 2•3 minutes.

6. Season with salt and pepper to taste.

7. Serve the chicken and green bean stir•fry over the cooked brown rice.

This stir•fry is a great option for weight loss because it's high in protein from the chicken, packed with fiber and nutrients from the green beans, and uses a light, flavorful sauce. Serving it over brown rice provides complex carbs to keep you feeling full and satisfied.

89. Roasted Eggplant and Tomato

Ingredient:

- 1 large eggplant, cut into 1•inch cubes
- 2 cups cherry or grape tomatoes, halved
- 3 tbsp olive oil
- 2 cloves garlic, minced
- 1 tsp dried oregano
- 1/2 tsp salt
- 1/4 tsp black pepper
- 2 tbsp balsamic glaze (or balsamic vinegar)
- 2 tbsp chopped fresh basil

Instructions:

1. Preheat your oven to 400°F (200°C).

2. In a large bowl, toss the cubed eggplant and halved tomatoes with the olive oil, garlic, oregano, salt, and black pepper until everything is well coated.

3. Spread the eggplant and tomato mixture in a single layer on a large baking sheet lined with parchment paper.

4. Roast the vegetables in the preheated oven for 25•30 minutes, stirring halfway, until the eggplant is tender and the tomatoes are softened and starting to burst.

5. Remove the roasted eggplant and tomatoes from the oven and transfer them to a serving dish.

6. Drizzle the balsamic glaze (or balsamic vinegar) over the top and sprinkle with the chopped fresh basil.

7. Serve the roasted eggplant and tomato dish warm or at room temperature.

This simple yet flavorful roasted eggplant and tomato dish makes a great side or can be served as a light main course. The balsamic glaze and fresh basil add a delicious finishing touch.

You can also toss the roasted vegetables with cooked pasta, quinoa, or serve them over a bed of greens for a more substantial meal.

90. Spicy Tofu Stir•Fry

Ingredient:

• 1 block (14 oz) extra•firm tofu, pressed and cubed
• 2 tbsp vegetable oil
• 2 cloves garlic, minced
• 1 tbsp grated ginger
• 1 red bell pepper, sliced
• 1 cup broccoli florets
• 2 cups baby spinach
• 2 tbsp soy sauce
• 1 tbsp rice vinegar
• 1•2 tsp chili garlic sauce (or to taste)
• 1 tsp sesame oil
• Salt and pepper to taste
• Chopped green onions and sesame seeds for garnish

Instructions:

1. In a large skillet or wok, heat the vegetable oil over medium•high heat. Add the cubed tofu and cook for 5•7 minutes, turning occasionally, until lightly browned on all sides. Transfer tofu to a plate.

2. In the same skillet, add the garlic and ginger. Cook for 1 minute until fragrant.

3. Add the sliced bell pepper and broccoli florets. Stir•fry for 3•4 minutes until vegetables are crisp•tender.

4. Add the cooked tofu back to the skillet. Pour in the soy sauce, rice vinegar, and chili garlic sauce. Toss everything together and cook for 2•3 minutes.

5. Stir in the baby spinach and sesame oil. Cook for 1 minute until the spinach is wilted.

6. Season with salt and pepper to taste.

7. Serve the spicy tofu stir•fry hot, garnished with chopped green onions and sesame seeds.

Enjoy this flavorful and nutritious spicy tofu stir•fry! The combination of crispy tofu, fresh veggies, and a spicy•sweet sauce makes for a delicious meatless meal.

91. Cottage Cheese with Sliced Peaches

Ingredient:

- 1 cup low•fat or non•fat cottage cheese
- 1 medium peach, sliced
- 1 tsp honey (optional)
- Cinnamon (optional)

Instructions:

1. Spoon the cottage cheese into a bowl or plate.

2. Arrange the sliced peaches on top of the cottage cheese.

3. Drizzle the honey over the top, if using. Sprinkle with a dash of cinnamon, if desired.

That's it! This simple dish provides a nice balance of protein, carbs, and healthy fats to keep you feeling full and satisfied.

The cottage cheese is a great source of lean protein, which can help support muscle growth and maintenance during weight loss. The peaches add natural sweetness and fiber, which can help regulate blood sugar levels and digestion.

This is a quick, easy, and nutritious snack or light meal that's perfect for young men looking to lose weight in a healthy way. The combination of cottage cheese and fruit makes it a filling and satisfying option.

92. Grilled Chicken and Veggie Skewers

Ingredient:

• 1 lb boneless, skinless chicken breasts, cut into 1·inch cubes
• 1 red bell pepper, cut into 1·inch pieces
• 1 zucchini, cut into 1·inch pieces
• 1 red onion, cut into 1·inch pieces
• 2 tbsp olive oil
• 2 tsp dried oregano
• 1 tsp garlic powder
• 1/2 tsp salt
• 1/4 tsp black pepper

Instructions:

1. Preheat grill or grill pan to medium·high heat.

2. In a large bowl, toss the chicken, bell pepper, zucchini, and onion with the olive oil, oregano, garlic powder, salt, and pepper until everything is evenly coated.

3. Thread the chicken and vegetables onto skewers, alternating the ingredients.

4. Grill the skewers for 12·15 minutes, turning occasionally, until the chicken is cooked through and the vegetables are tender.

5. Serve the grilled chicken and veggie skewers immediately.

This dish is perfect for weight loss for a few reasons:

• Grilled chicken is a lean protein that will help keep you feeling full and satisfied.
• The vegetables add fiber, vitamins, and minerals without a lot of calories.
• Grilling the ingredients adds great flavor without needing to use a lot of oil or sauces.
• The skewer format makes for a fun, easy·to·eat meal.

Serve the skewers with a side of roasted potatoes or a fresh salad for a complete, balanced meal. This is a delicious and nutritious option for young men looking to lose weight in a healthy way.

93. Mango and Avocado Salad

Ingredient:

- 2 ripe mangoes, peeled and diced
- 1 ripe avocado, diced
- 1/2 red onion, thinly sliced
- 1 jalapeño, seeded and minced (optional)
- 1/4 cup chopped fresh cilantro
- 2 tbsp lime juice
- 1 tbsp olive oil
- 1/4 tsp salt
- 1/4 tsp black pepper

Instructions:

1. In a large bowl, gently combine the diced mango, avocado, red onion, and jalapeño (if using).

2. Add the chopped cilantro, lime juice, olive oil, salt, and black pepper. Toss everything together until well mixed.

3. Taste and adjust seasoning as needed, adding more lime juice, salt, or pepper to your preference.

4. Serve the mango and avocado salad chilled or at room temperature.

This salad makes a refreshing and flavorful side dish or light main course. The sweet mango pairs beautifully with the creamy avocado, while the red onion, jalapeño, and lime juice add a nice contrast of flavors and textures.

You can customize the salad by adding other ingredients like cherry tomatoes, crumbled feta or queso fresco, toasted nuts, or a drizzle of honey. Enjoy this vibrant and healthy mango and avocado salad!

94. Cauliflower and Chickpea Curry

Ingredient:

- 1 tbsp olive oil
- 1 onion, diced
- 3 cloves garlic, minced
- 1 tbsp grated fresh ginger
- 2 tsp garam masala
- 1 tsp ground cumin
- 1 tsp ground coriander
- 1/4 tsp cayenne pepper (optional)
- 1 head cauliflower, cut into florets
- 1 (15 oz) can chickpeas, drained and rinsed
- 1 (14 oz) can diced tomatoes
- 1 cup low·sodium vegetable or chicken broth
- 1 cup light coconut milk
- Salt and black pepper to taste
- Chopped cilantro for serving

Instructions:

1. In a large pot or Dutch oven, heat the olive oil over medium heat. Add the onion and cook for 5 minutes until translucent.

2. Add the garlic, ginger, garam masala, cumin, coriander, and cayenne (if using). Cook for 1 minute until fragrant.

3. Stir in the cauliflower florets, chickpeas, diced tomatoes, broth, and coconut milk. Bring to a simmer.

4. Reduce heat to medium·low and let the curry simmer for 15·20 minutes, until the cauliflower is tender.

5. Season with salt and pepper to taste. Serve the curry over basmati rice or with naan bread. Top with chopped cilantro.

This curry is a great option for weight loss because it's packed with fiber, protein, and nutrients from the cauliflower and chickpeas. The coconut milk provides a creamy texture without a lot of added fat or calories. It's a flavorful, satisfying dish that will keep you feeling full.

95. Baked Zucchini Chips

Ingredient:

• 2 medium zucchinis, sliced into 1/4•inch thick rounds
• 1 tbsp olive oil
• 1/2 tsp garlic powder
• 1/2 tsp onion powder
• 1/4 tsp salt
• 1/4 tsp black pepper

Instructions:

1. Preheat oven to 400°F. Line two baking sheets with parchment paper.

2. In a large bowl, toss the zucchini slices with the olive oil, garlic powder, onion powder, salt, and pepper until evenly coated.

3. Arrange the zucchini slices in a single layer on the prepared baking sheets, making sure they are not overlapping.

4. Bake for 12•15 minutes, flipping the slices halfway through, until the edges are lightly browned and crispy.

5. Remove from oven and let cool for 5 minutes before serving.

These baked zucchini chips make a great healthy snack option for weight loss for a few reasons:

• Zucchini is low in calories and high in fiber, which can help keep you feeling full.
• Baking the zucchini slices instead of frying them cuts down significantly on fat and calories.
• The simple seasoning adds flavor without a lot of extra calories or sodium.

Zucchini chips are a great alternative to potato chips or other high•calorie snacks. They provide a satisfying crunch and can curb cravings for something salty and crispy. Enjoy them on their own or with a healthy dip like Greek yogurt or hummus.

96. Seared Tuna with Sesame Seeds

Ingredient:

• 4 (4 oz) tuna steaks
• 2 tbsp sesame seeds
• 1 tbsp olive oil
• 1 tbsp low•sodium soy sauce
• 1 tsp rice vinegar
• 1 tsp honey
• 1/2 tsp sesame oil
• 1/4 tsp red pepper flakes (optional)
• Salt and black pepper to taste

Instructions:

1. Pat the tuna steaks dry with paper towels and season both sides with salt and pepper.

2. In a shallow bowl, coat the tuna steaks evenly with the sesame seeds, pressing gently to help them adhere.

3. Heat the olive oil in a large skillet over high heat.

4. When the oil is hot, add the tuna steaks and sear for 1•2 minutes per side, until the outside is lightly browned but the inside is still pink and rare.

5. In a small bowl, whisk together the soy sauce, rice vinegar, honey, sesame oil, and red pepper flakes (if using).

6. Drizzle the sauce over the seared tuna steaks and serve immediately.

This seared tuna dish is an excellent option for weight loss for a few reasons:

• Tuna is a lean, high•protein fish that can help keep you feeling full and satisfied.
• The sesame seeds add a nice crunch and nutty flavor without a lot of extra calories.
• The simple sauce provides flavor without adding a lot of sugar or sodium.

Serve the tuna with a side of roasted vegetables or a fresh salad for a complete, balanced meal. This is a delicious and nutritious option for young men looking to lose weight in a healthy way.

97. Roasted Fennel and Carrots

Ingredient:

- 2 fennel bulbs, trimmed and cut into 1·inch wedges
- 6 medium carrots, peeled and cut into 1·inch pieces
- 2 tbsp olive oil
- 1 tsp dried thyme
- 1 tsp ground cumin
- 1/2 tsp salt
- 1/4 tsp black pepper
- 2 tbsp chopped fresh parsley

Instructions:

1. Preheat your oven to 400°F (200°C).

2. In a large bowl, combine the fennel wedges and carrot pieces. Drizzle with the olive oil and sprinkle with the dried thyme, cumin, salt, and black pepper. Toss everything together until the vegetables are evenly coated.

3. Spread the seasoned fennel and carrots in a single layer on a large baking sheet lined with parchment paper.

4. Roast the vegetables in the preheated oven for 25·30 minutes, flipping them halfway through, until they are tender and lightly browned.

5. Remove the roasted fennel and carrots from the oven and transfer them to a serving dish.

6. Sprinkle the chopped fresh parsley over the top and serve immediately.

This simple roasted fennel and carrots dish makes a great side or can be enjoyed as a light main course. The fennel and carrots become sweet and caramelized in the oven, and the herbs and spices add a delicious depth of flavor.

98. Chicken and Bell Pepper Stir•Fry

Ingredient:

• 1 lb boneless, skinless chicken breasts, cut into 1•inch pieces
• 2 tbsp low•sodium soy sauce
• 1 tbsp rice vinegar
• 1 tsp sesame oil
• 1 tbsp olive oil
• 1 red bell pepper, sliced
• 1 yellow bell pepper, sliced
• 1 cup sliced mushrooms
• 3 cloves garlic, minced
• 1 tbsp grated fresh ginger
• 2 cups cooked brown rice, for serving

For the Sauce:
• 2 tbsp low•sodium soy sauce
• 1 tbsp rice vinegar
• 1 tsp honey
• 1/2 tsp cornstarch
• 1/4 tsp red pepper flakes (optional)

Instructions:

1. In a small bowl, whisk together the 2 tbsp soy sauce, 1 tbsp rice vinegar, and 1 tsp sesame oil. Add the chicken and toss to coat. Let marinate for 15 minutes.

2. In another small bowl, whisk together the sauce ingredients (2 tbsp soy sauce, 1 tbsp rice vinegar, honey, cornstarch, and red pepper flakes if using).

3. Heat the olive oil in a large skillet or wok over high heat. Add the chicken and stir•fry for 3•4 minutes until lightly browned.

4. Add the bell peppers, mushrooms, garlic, and ginger. Stir•fry for 4•5 minutes until the vegetables are tender•crisp.

5. Pour in the sauce and cook for 1•2 minutes, stirring constantly, until the sauce has thickened. Serve the chicken and vegetable stir•fry over the cooked brown rice.

This stir•fry is a great option for weight loss because it's high in protein from the chicken, packed with fiber and nutrients from the vegetables, and uses a light, flavorful sauce. Serving it over brown rice provides complex carbs to keep you feeling full and satisfied.

99. Lentil and Spinach Salad

Ingredient:

• 1 cup cooked lentils, cooled
• 4 cups baby spinach leaves
• 1 cup cherry tomatoes, halved
• 1/2 cucumber, diced
• 1/4 red onion, thinly sliced
• 2 tbsp crumbled feta cheese
• 2 tbsp olive oil
• 1 tbsp red wine vinegar
• 1 tsp Dijon mustard
• 1 tsp honey
• Salt and black pepper to taste

Instructions:

1. In a large bowl, combine the cooked lentils, spinach, tomatoes, cucumber, and red onion.

2. In a small bowl, whisk together the olive oil, red wine vinegar, Dijon mustard, and honey. Season with salt and pepper.

3. Drizzle the dressing over the lentil and spinach salad and toss gently to coat.

4. Top the salad with the crumbled feta cheese.

This lentil and spinach salad is an excellent choice for weight loss for several reasons:

• Lentils are a great source of plant•based protein and fiber, which can help keep you feeling full.
• Spinach is low in calories but packed with vitamins, minerals, and antioxidants.
• The fresh vegetables add crunch, flavor, and more fiber.
• The simple vinaigrette dressing provides flavor without a lot of extra calories or fat.

This salad makes for a satisfying, nutrient•dense meal or side dish. The combination of protein, fiber, and healthy fats will help support weight loss goals. Feel free to add grilled chicken or hard•boiled eggs for extra protein if desired.

100. Stuffed Cabbage Rolls

Ingredient:

• 1 medium head green cabbage
• 1 lb lean ground turkey or ground chicken
• 1 cup cooked brown rice
• 1 onion, finely chopped
• 2 cloves garlic, minced
• 1 tsp dried oregano
• 1/2 tsp dried basil
• 1/4 tsp red pepper flakes (optional)
• Salt and black pepper to taste
• 1 (15 oz) can tomato sauce
• 1/4 cup low•sodium chicken or vegetable broth

Instructions:

1. Bring a large pot of water to a boil. Using a paring knife, carefully cut out the core of the cabbage. Place the whole cabbage head in the boiling water and cook for 3•5 minutes until the outer leaves are softened. Remove the cabbage and let cool slightly.

2. Carefully peel off the softened cabbage leaves, keeping them intact. You should get about 12•14 leaves.

3. In a large bowl, mix together the ground turkey/chicken, cooked rice, onion, garlic, oregano, basil, red pepper flakes (if using), and salt and pepper.

4. Place about 2•3 tablespoons of the filling onto the center of each cabbage leaf. Fold the sides of the leaf over the filling, then roll up tightly.

5. Arrange the stuffed cabbage rolls seam•side down in a baking dish. Pour the tomato sauce and broth over the top.

6. Cover the dish with foil and bake at 375°F for 45•55 minutes, until the cabbage is tender and the filling is cooked through.

These stuffed cabbage rolls are a great option for weight loss because they are low in calories and high in protein, fiber, and nutrients. The lean ground turkey or chicken provides a filling protein source, while the cabbage and rice add complex carbs and fiber to keep you feeling satisfied. Enjoy this hearty, comforting dish as part of a healthy, balanced diet.

101. Grilled Vegetable Salad

Ingredient:

• 1 zucchini, sliced lengthwise into 1/2•inch thick strips
• 1 yellow squash, sliced lengthwise into 1/2•inch thick strips
• 1 red bell pepper, cut into 1•inch pieces
• 1 red onion, sliced into 1/2•inch thick rounds
• 2 tbsp olive oil
• 1 tsp dried oregano
• 1/2 tsp garlic powder
• 1/4 tsp salt
• 1/4 tsp black pepper
• 4 cups mixed greens
• 1 tbsp balsamic vinegar
• 2 tbsp crumbled feta cheese (optional)

Instructions:

1. Preheat grill or grill pan to medium•high heat.

2. In a large bowl, toss the zucchini, yellow squash, bell pepper, and onion with the olive oil, oregano, garlic powder, salt, and pepper until evenly coated.

3. Grill the vegetables for 4•6 minutes per side, until tender and lightly charred. Remove the vegetables from the grill and let cool slightly. Chop the grilled vegetables into bite•sized pieces.

4. In a large salad bowl, combine the chopped grilled vegetables and mixed greens. Drizzle with the balsamic vinegar and toss to coat. Top the salad with the crumbled feta cheese, if using.

This grilled vegetable salad is an excellent choice for weight loss for a few reasons:

• The grilled vegetables provide fiber, vitamins, and minerals without a lot of calories.
• The mixed greens add more fiber and nutrients to keep you feeling full.
• The balsamic vinegar dressing provides flavor without a lot of added sugar or fat.
• The optional feta cheese adds a creamy, tangy element with a small amount of healthy fat.

This salad makes for a satisfying, nutrient•dense meal or side dish. Feel free to add grilled chicken or chickpeas for extra protein if desired. The combination of vegetables, greens, and a light dressing makes this a great option for young men looking to lose weight in a healthy way.

102. Roasted Acorn Squash

Ingredient:

• 1 medium acorn squash, halved and seeded
• 1 tbsp olive oil
• 1 tsp maple syrup (optional)
• 1/2 tsp ground cinnamon
• 1/4 tsp ground nutmeg
• Salt and black pepper to taste

Instructions:
1. Preheat oven to 400°F. Line a baking sheet with parchment paper.

2. Place the acorn squash halves cut•side up on the prepared baking sheet.

3. Brush the squash halves with the olive oil. If using, drizzle the maple syrup over the top.

4. Sprinkle the cinnamon, nutmeg, salt, and pepper evenly over the squash.

5. Roast for 40•50 minutes, until the squash is very tender when pierced with a fork.

6. Remove from oven and let cool for 5 minutes.

7. Scoop out the roasted squash flesh and serve.

Acorn squash is an excellent choice for weight loss for a few reasons:

• It's low in calories but high in fiber, which can help keep you feeling full and satisfied.
• The natural sweetness means you don't need to add a lot of extra sugar or butter to make it taste good.
• The vitamins, minerals, and antioxidants in squash provide important nutrients without a lot of calories.

This simple roasted acorn squash recipe allows the natural flavors of the squash to shine. The cinnamon and nutmeg add warmth and depth without a lot of added calories. Enjoy the squash on its own or use it as a side dish to accompany a lean protein like grilled chicken or fish.

103. Spicy Shrimp and Veggie Stir•Fry

Ingredient:

• 1 lb raw shrimp, peeled and deveined
• 2 tbsp low•sodium soy sauce
• 1 tbsp rice vinegar
• 1 tsp sesame oil
• 1 tbsp olive oil
• 3 cloves garlic, minced
• 1 tbsp grated fresh ginger
• 1 red bell pepper, sliced
• 1 cup broccoli florets
• 1 cup snow peas
• 2 cups cooked brown rice, for serving
• 1•2 tsp Sriracha or other hot sauce (optional)
• Chopped green onions for garnish

Instructions:

1. In a medium bowl, combine the shrimp, soy sauce, rice vinegar, and sesame oil. Toss to coat and let marinate for 15 minutes.

2. Heat the olive oil in a large skillet or wok over high heat.

3. Add the garlic and ginger and cook for 1 minute until fragrant.

4. Add the marinated shrimp and stir•fry for 2•3 minutes until the shrimp start to turn pink.

5. Add the bell pepper, broccoli, and snow peas. Stir•fry for 3•4 minutes until the vegetables are tender•crisp.

6. If using, stir in the Sriracha or hot sauce to taste.

7. Serve the spicy shrimp and veggie stir•fry over the cooked brown rice, garnished with chopped green onions.

The Sriracha or other hot sauce is optional, but it can add a nice kick of flavor and spice. Adjust the amount to your personal preference. This dish makes for a quick, easy, and nutritious meal that's perfect for young men looking to lose weight in a healthy way.

104. Eggplant and Chickpea Stew

Ingredient:

- 1 medium eggplant, cut into 1•inch cubes
- 1 tbsp olive oil
- 1 onion, diced
- 3 cloves garlic, minced
- 1 tsp ground cumin
- 1 tsp paprika
- 1/4 tsp cayenne pepper (optional)
- 1 (15 oz) can chickpeas, drained and rinsed
- 1 (14.5 oz) can diced tomatoes
- 1 cup low•sodium vegetable or chicken broth
- 1 tbsp tomato paste
- 1 tsp dried oregano
- Salt and black pepper to taste
- Chopped parsley for serving

Instructions:

1. In a large pot or Dutch oven, heat the olive oil over medium heat. Add the eggplant cubes and cook for 5•7 minutes, stirring occasionally, until lightly browned.

2. Add the onion and cook for 3•4 minutes until translucent. Stir in the garlic, cumin, paprika, and cayenne (if using). Cook for 1 minute until fragrant.

3. Add the chickpeas, diced tomatoes, broth, tomato paste, and oregano. Stir to combine.

4. Bring the stew to a simmer and let it cook for 20•25 minutes, until the eggplant is very tender.

5. Season with salt and pepper to taste.

6. Serve the eggplant and chickpea stew warm, garnished with chopped parsley.

Enjoy this hearty, vegetable•packed stew on its own or serve it over a small portion of whole grain rice or quinoa for a more substantial meal. It's a delicious and nutritious option for young men looking to lose weight in a healthy way.

105. Greek Yogurt with Chia Seeds

Ingredient:

• 1 cup plain Greek yogurt
• 1 tbsp chia seeds
• 1 tsp honey (optional)
• 1/2 cup fresh berries (such as blueberries, raspberries, or strawberries)

Instructions:

1. In a small bowl, stir together the Greek yogurt and chia seeds until well combined.

2. If desired, drizzle the honey over the top of the yogurt and chia seed mixture.

3. Top with the fresh berries.

That's it! This simple snack takes just a few minutes to prepare.

This Greek yogurt with chia seeds is an excellent choice for weight loss for several reasons:

• Greek yogurt is high in protein, which can help keep you feeling full and satisfied.

• Chia seeds are a great source of fiber, healthy fats, and antioxidants.

• The fresh berries add natural sweetness, fiber, and important vitamins and minerals.

• The optional honey provides a touch of sweetness without a lot of added sugar.

The combination of protein, fiber, and healthy fats in this snack makes it very filling and nutritious. It can help curb hunger and cravings between meals, supporting your weight loss goals.

This is a versatile snack that can be enjoyed on its own or paired with whole grain crackers or a small handful of nuts for a more substantial option. It's a quick, easy, and delicious way for young men to incorporate more healthy foods into their diet.

106. Baked Chicken with Herbs

Ingredient:

• 4 boneless, skinless chicken breasts
• 2 tbsp olive oil
• 1 tsp dried thyme
• 1 tsp dried rosemary
• 1 tsp dried oregano
• 1/2 tsp garlic powder
• 1/4 tsp salt
• 1/4 tsp black pepper
• Lemon wedges for serving (optional)

Instructions:

1. Preheat oven to 400°F. Line a baking sheet with parchment paper.

2. Pat the chicken breasts dry with paper towels and place them on the prepared baking sheet.

3. In a small bowl, mix together the olive oil, thyme, rosemary, oregano, garlic powder, salt, and pepper.

4. Brush the herb mixture evenly over the top of the chicken breasts, making sure to coat them completely.

5. Bake for 25·30 minutes, until the chicken is cooked through and reaches an internal temperature of 165°F. Serve the baked chicken immediately, with lemon wedges on the side if desired.

This baked chicken dish is an excellent option for weight loss for a few reasons:

• Chicken breast is a lean protein that will help keep you feeling full and satisfied.
• The simple herb seasoning adds tons of flavor without a lot of extra calories or fat.
• Baking the chicken is a healthier cooking method compared to frying.
• Serving it with lemon wedges provides a bright, fresh flavor boost without needing to use heavy sauces.

This baked chicken pairs perfectly with roasted vegetables or a fresh salad for a complete, balanced meal. It's an easy, delicious, and nutritious option for young men looking to lose weight in a healthy way.

107. Grilled Tilapia with Veggies

Ingredient:

• 4 tilapia fillets (about 1 lb total)
• 2 tbsp olive oil
• 1 tsp lemon pepper seasoning
• 1 zucchini, sliced into 1/2•inch rounds
• 1 yellow squash, sliced into 1/2•inch rounds
• 1 red bell pepper, sliced into strips
• 1 red onion, sliced into 1/2•inch rounds
• 2 tbsp balsamic vinegar
• Salt and black pepper to taste
• Lemon wedges for serving

Instructions:

1. Preheat grill or grill pan to medium•high heat.

2. Brush the tilapia fillets with 1 tbsp of the olive oil and sprinkle with the lemon pepper seasoning.

3. In a large bowl, toss the zucchini, yellow squash, bell pepper, and onion with the remaining 1 tbsp olive oil and balsamic vinegar. Season with salt and pepper.

4. Grill the tilapia for 4•5 minutes per side, until opaque and flaky.

5. Grill the vegetable slices for 3•4 minutes per side, until tender and lightly charred. Serve the grilled tilapia fillets with the grilled vegetables. Squeeze fresh lemon juice over the top.

This grilled tilapia and vegetable dish is an excellent choice for weight loss for several reasons:

• Tilapia is a lean, protein•rich fish that will help keep you feeling full.
• The grilled vegetables add fiber, vitamins, and minerals without a lot of calories.
• The simple seasoning and balsamic vinegar provide flavor without relying on high•calorie sauces or dressings.
• Grilling the ingredients adds great taste while keeping the dish low in fat.

Serve this meal with a side of roasted potatoes or a fresh green salad for a complete, balanced dinner. The combination of protein, vegetables, and healthy fats will support your weight loss goals in a delicious and nutritious way.

108. Broccoli and Quinoa Salad

Ingredient:

• 1 cup cooked quinoa, cooled
• 2 cups chopped broccoli florets
• 1/2 cup diced cucumber
• 1/4 cup diced red onion
• 2 tbsp chopped fresh parsley
• 2 tbsp olive oil
• 1 tbsp lemon juice
• 1 tsp Dijon mustard
• 1/4 tsp salt
• 1/4 tsp black pepper
• 2 tbsp crumbled feta cheese (optional)

Instructions:

1. In a large bowl, combine the cooked quinoa, broccoli, cucumber, red onion, and parsley.

2. In a small bowl, whisk together the olive oil, lemon juice, Dijon mustard, salt, and pepper.

3. Pour the dressing over the quinoa and vegetable mixture and toss gently to coat.

4. Top the salad with the crumbled feta cheese, if using.

5. Refrigerate the salad for at least 30 minutes to allow the flavors to meld.

This broccoli and quinoa salad is an excellent choice for weight loss for several reasons:

• Quinoa is a high•protein, high•fiber grain that will help keep you feeling full.
• Broccoli is low in calories but packed with fiber, vitamins, and minerals.
• The fresh vegetables add crunch, flavor, and more fiber.
• The simple lemon•Dijon dressing provides flavor without a lot of extra calories or fat.
• The optional feta cheese adds a creamy, tangy element with a small amount of healthy fat.

This salad makes for a satisfying, nutrient•dense meal or side dish. The combination of protein, fiber, and healthy fats will support your weight loss goals in a delicious and nutritious way. Feel free to add grilled chicken or chickpeas for extra protein if desired.

109. Roasted Sweet Potato and Black Beans

Ingredient:

- 2 medium sweet potatoes, peeled and cubed
- 1 tbsp olive oil
- 1 tsp chili powder
- 1/2 tsp ground cumin
- 1/4 tsp garlic powder
- Salt and black pepper to taste
- 1 (15 oz) can black beans, drained and rinsed
- 1 cup frozen corn kernels
- 2 tbsp chopped fresh cilantro
- 1 tbsp lime juice

Instructions:

1. Preheat oven to 400°F. Line a baking sheet with parchment paper.

2. In a large bowl, toss the cubed sweet potatoes with the olive oil, chili powder, cumin, garlic powder, salt, and pepper until evenly coated.

3. Spread the seasoned sweet potato cubes in a single layer on the prepared baking sheet.

4. Roast for 20•25 minutes, flipping halfway, until the sweet potatoes are tender and lightly browned.

5. Remove the sweet potatoes from the oven and transfer to a large bowl. Add the black beans, frozen corn, cilantro, and lime juice. Toss to combine.

6. Serve the roasted sweet potato and black bean mixture warm.

This dish is an excellent option for weight loss for several reasons:

- Sweet potatoes are high in fiber, vitamins, and complex carbs to keep you feeling full.
- Black beans provide plant•based protein and fiber.
- The simple seasonings add flavor without a lot of extra calories or sodium.
- It's a versatile dish that can be enjoyed on its own or served over quinoa or brown rice.

The combination of roasted sweet potatoes, black beans, and fresh cilantro and lime makes for a flavorful, nutrient•dense meal that's perfect for young men looking to lose weight in a healthy way. Adjust the spices to your taste preferences.

110. Cucumber and Yogurt Dip

Ingredient:

• 1 cup plain Greek yogurt
• 1 cup grated cucumber, squeezed dry
• 2 tbsp chopped fresh dill
• 1 tbsp lemon juice
• 1 clove garlic, minced
• 1/4 tsp salt
• 1/4 tsp black pepper

Serve with:
• Carrot sticks
• Celery sticks
• Whole grain pita chips or crackers

Instructions:

1. In a medium bowl, stir together the Greek yogurt, grated cucumber, dill, lemon juice, garlic, salt, and pepper until well combined.

2. Cover and refrigerate the dip for at least 30 minutes to allow the flavors to meld.

3. Serve the cucumber yogurt dip chilled, with carrot sticks, celery sticks, pita chips, or other crunchy dippers.

This cucumber yogurt dip is an excellent snack option for weight loss for a few reasons:

• Greek yogurt is high in protein, which can help keep you feeling full.
• Cucumbers are low in calories but high in fiber and water content, making them very filling.
• The simple seasoning adds flavor without a lot of extra calories or fat.

Pairing the dip with fresh veggies or whole grain crackers provides a satisfying, nutrient•dense snack. The protein, fiber, and hydration from the yogurt and cucumbers can help curb hunger and cravings between meals.

This dip is easy to make and can be kept in the fridge for up to 5 days, making it a convenient and healthy snack option for young men looking to lose weight.

111. Grilled Chicken Breast with Salsa

Ingredient:

- 4 boneless, skinless chicken breasts
- 1 tbsp olive oil
- 1 tsp chili powder
- 1/2 tsp garlic powder
- 1/4 tsp salt
- 1/4 tsp black pepper

For the Salsa:
- 1 cup diced tomatoes
- 1/2 cup diced red onion
- 1/4 cup chopped fresh cilantro
- 1 jalapeño, seeded and finely chopped (optional)
- 1 tbsp lime juice
- 1/4 tsp salt

Instructions:

1. Preheat grill or grill pan to medium•high heat.

2. In a small bowl, mix together the olive oil, chili powder, garlic powder, salt, and pepper. Rub this seasoning mixture all over the chicken breasts.

3. Grill the chicken for 5•7 minutes per side, until cooked through and no longer pink in the center.

4. While the chicken is grilling, prepare the salsa. In a medium bowl, combine the diced tomatoes, red onion, cilantro, jalapeño (if using), lime juice, and salt. Stir to mix well. Serve the grilled chicken breasts topped with the fresh tomato salsa.

This grilled chicken and salsa dish is an excellent choice for weight loss for a few reasons:

- Grilled chicken breast is a lean protein that will help keep you feeling full and satisfied.
- The fresh salsa adds flavor, vitamins, and fiber without a lot of extra calories.
- The simple seasoning on the chicken provides taste without relying on high•calorie sauces or dressings.

Serve this dish with a side of roasted vegetables or a fresh green salad for a complete, balanced meal. The combination of protein, vegetables, and healthy fats will support your weight loss goals in a delicious and nutritious way.

Congratulations on reaching the end of ***"Cookbook for Weight Loss Young Men: Tasty, Low-Calorie Dishes to Boost Your Weight Loss Journey."*** You've embarked on a significant step towards achieving a healthier, fitter, and more energetic version of yourself. Throughout this book, we've explored a diverse range of recipes designed to make your weight loss journey not just effective, but also enjoyable and sustainable.

By incorporating these delicious, low-calorie meals into your daily routine, you've learned that healthy eating doesn't have to be a chore or bland. Instead, it can be a delightful and rewarding experience that fuels your body and satisfies your taste buds. These recipes are not just about losing weight; they are about building lifelong habits that promote overall well-being.

Remember, the journey to a healthier you is a marathon, not a sprint. It's about making consistent, mindful choices that align with your goals. Continue to experiment with the recipes, adapt them to your preferences, and most importantly, enjoy the process. Healthy eating is a lifestyle, and with the knowledge and skills you've gained, you're well-equipped to maintain this lifestyle long after you've achieved your weight loss goals.

In addition to the recipes, the tips and strategies provided in this book are tools you can use to navigate the challenges that come with maintaining a healthy diet. From meal prepping and smart grocery shopping to understanding nutritional information, you've acquired valuable skills that will serve you well beyond the kitchen.

As you continue your journey, remember that progress is more important than perfection. Celebrate your successes, no matter how small, and learn from any setbacks. Surround yourself with supportive people who encourage your healthy habits, and don't hesitate to revisit this book whenever you need inspiration or motivation.

Thank you for allowing this cookbook to be a part of your weight loss journey. We hope it has been a helpful and enjoyable resource, guiding you toward your goals with flavorful, nourishing meals. Here's to your continued success, health, and happiness. Keep cooking, keep striving, and most importantly, keep taking care of yourself.

Happy cooking, and best of luck on your journey to a healthier you!